Saliva and Dental Health

Clinical implications of saliva and salivary
stimulation for better dental health in the 1990s

Report of a Consensus Workshop held at Ashford Castle,
Co. Mayo, Ireland, July 2–5, 1989

Edited by

Professor W. M. Edgar
School of Dentistry
University of Liverpool

Professor D. M. O'Mullane
Department of Preventive Dentistry
University College, Cork

1990

Published by the British Dental Association
64 Wimpole Street, London W1M 8AL

First Edition 1990

ISBN 0 904588 30 0

Typeset, printed and bound in Great Britain by
Latimer Trend and Company Ltd, Plymouth

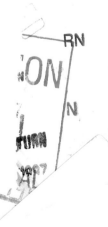
WITHDRAWN FROM STOCK
The University of Liverpool
C 1996

Foreword

Few people outside the field of oral research realise the fascinating range of diverse properties and functions of saliva, or its contributions to the prevention of disease, the promotion of comfort, general health and the pleasures of eating. These proceedings, of the conference at Ashford Castle, collect together valuable summaries of work on saliva during the last few years, and update it with many more recent results and accounts of work still in progress.

The fall in dental caries over the last two decades has tended to induce some complacency and to convey the impression that the caries problem is solved and that further research on saliva should now have a low priority. This attitude overlooks several facts. First, the decline seems now to have stabilised, leaving about half the previous incidence still requiring attention. Secondly, the decline has occurred only in westernised countries and the reverse—an increase in caries—has been reported in the developing countries as the result of greater availability of sugar and, in some cases, its introduction into the diet for the first time. It is also possible that because fluoride, in toothpaste, is the often accepted cause of this decline, intensive research on the effects of fluoride has diverted interest away from saliva, the other great protector of the teeth and the oral structures generally. This conference is therefore all the more welcome in drawing attention to the importance of saliva and its potential for preventing caries.

The conference has also tackled in a rational way the problems of xerostomia—problems which are increasing rather than declining as the proportion of the population in the later stages of life increases. It is reassuring to see the evidence that xerostomia is not a result of old age itself but is usually iatrogenic and therefore potentially preventable. It is also encouraging to see the results of a double-blind clinical trial on pilocarpine showing that, as a saliva stimulant, it is a promising treatment in many cases, without undue side effects.

Several original, or very new, suggestions are made. One is that saliva flow-rates should be routinely measured by dentists as a measure of oral health in much the same way as blood pressure is measured by the physician as a check on general fitness. This is an idea well worth considering, although the list of the many factors that would have to be controlled to ensure meaningful results is somewhat off-putting! Perhaps more practicable, if of more restricted importance, is the suggestion of deciding on an international standard stimulus (such as 5% citric acid) to increase the validity of comparing different sets of results.

In discussing the effects of the low concentrations of sodium, chloride and glucose in saliva compared with plasma, it is pointed out that this prevents adaptation of the taste buds thus increasing their sensitivity to salt and sweet tastes. Whether this is the 'probable reason' for these low concentrations, as stated, is a nice philosophical point.

Several contributors discuss, perhaps, the most important properties of saliva from the caries point of view, namely, its buffering power and its saturation with calcium phosphate and how these factors increase as the pH is raised and are reduced when the pH falls sufficiently. An important gap in our knowledge is also mentioned: does the pH of plaque fall during the eating of a carbohydrate meal or only after the last mouthful has been swallowed and the saliva flow and its buffering power are greatly reduced? Clearly, the preventive measures required to maintain the saturation of the plaque with calcium phosphate during a meal differ (and are much more difficult to apply) from those required if unsaturation occurs only after eating is finished (as the limited data rather suggest).

Among the papers on xerostomia both simple and sophisticated methods of deciding whether a patient is suffering from a deficiency of gland tissue or an underfunctioning of surviving tissue are described. If the former, then saliva substitutes are needed and it is pointed out that more work is needed to define the exact properties (such as viscosity? lubrication?) substitutes would need to alleviate, more successfully than at present, the discomforts of xerostomia.

If there is functioning tissue, then eating a bulky diet would be expected to stimulate it, as it does in rats, but its value in human patients was considered by one author to be under-investigated. In a piece of work I carried out, in collaboration with one of the editors of these proceedings, it was shown that gum-chewing between meals by students resulted in raising unstimulated saliva flow-rates, especially among slow secretors—an effect still detectable several weeks after the gum-chewing had finished, which implies some structural effect on the glands (Jenkins GN, Edgar WM. *J Dent Res* 1989; **68**: 786–790. This suggests that exercising the salivary glands in other ways might increase their resulting flow. This may be clinically valuable because the results of a computer model, described later in this book, indicate that resting flow is a major factor controlling sugar clearance from the mouth. A practical difficulty is that those factors that increase sugar clearance, with its benefits, also increase the removal of protective substances like fluoride and a recommendation to meet this problem is made.

The concluding papers give us a peep into the future in which the application of genetic engineering and of the possibility of manipulation of the complicated secretory mechanisms of the salivary glands to improve their function is considered.

I hope and believe that this publication will sustain and extend the realisation of the multitude of valuable properties that saliva possesses and will encourage research workers to continue to fill the gaps in our knowledge of this unique biological fluid.

Professor G. Neil Jenkins
July, 1990

Preface

This book arises from a 2-day Consensus Meeting of selected, world-renowned experts on saliva and salivation who were gathered together under the auspices of the University of Cork and supported by the Wm Wrigley Jr Co. to discuss the role of saliva in dental health, and practical aspects of salivary stimulation for clinical dentistry, and especially preventive dentistry of the future. The programme was planned by Dr Colin Dawes, who also selected the participants.

The meeting was held in a magnificent castle in a beautiful corner of Ireland on the shores of Loch Corib, reputed to be one of the finest fishing lakes in the world. The meeting was chaired by two major figures in dental research, both of them having held the office of President of the International Association for Dental Research. It is particularly fitting that the chairman for the first day was an Irishman. Dr Bill Bowen, formerly at the Royal College of Surgeons of England, London, is now head of the Department of Dental Research, University of Rochester, USA. Dr Bowen recalled the Irish toast—'The health of the salmon to you: a long life, a full heart and a wet mouth'—and stressed that the purpose of the meeting was to report on how dental practitioners can help their patients by maintaining a wet mouth.

On the other hand, the chairman for the second day of the meeting, referred to the change in perspective of the profession concerning saliva—regarded as a hindrance to restorative techniques until relatively recently. Dr Ernest Newbrun of the University of California, San Francisco, and author of widely-used textbooks on cariology and fluorides, stressed the essential role of saliva in controlling the environment of the teeth, the benefits to be gained by stimulation and the problems experienced by patients with xerostomia.

The papers were presented in an informal manner allowing full and detailed discussion of each point raised, with the chairman taking pains to ensure that practical, clinical aspects were highlighted. The papers and discussion were taped, and the proceedings transcribed before being extensively edited. What remains is presented in this book, with the aim of summarising in a concise and practical way the present knowledge of saliva and its importance for dental health. It is aimed at the general dental practitioner in the interests of his or her continuing training and to promote the preventive aspects of salivary secretion and properties.

The list of contributors and the titles of their papers, together with other invited delegates, is shown overleaf. The papers formed the basis of the relevant chapters of this book, but points made by other contributors during the general discussion periods have been incorporated in the chapters, and the text has been extensively simplified and edited. The views expressed in this book do not, therefore, necessarily correspond with those of the presenters of the papers. Nevertheless, without their contributions, to act as a source and template, the chapters could not have been compiled, and the editors wish to express their gratitude for the generous help they have received from the contributors at all stages in the preparation of the book.

W. M. Edgar and D. M. O'Mullane
May, 1990

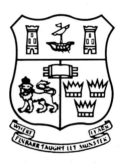

Coláiste na hOllscoile Corcaigh, Éire
University College Cork, Ireland

Contributors

Dr William H. Bowen, PhD, BDS, Professor and Chair, Department of Dental Research, University of Rochester, School of Medicine and Dentistry, Rochester, New York, USA.

Dr Colin Dawes, PhD, BSc, BDS, Professor of Oral Biology, Department of Oral Biology, University of Manitoba, Winnipeg, Manitoba, Canada. (Physiological factors influencing salivary flow rate and composition.)

Dr G. H. Dibdin, PhD, BSc, MSc, Research Scientist, Medical Research Council Dental Group, Dental School, University of Bristol, Bristol, UK.

Professor W. M. Edgar, PhD, BDS, BSc, DDSc, Professor of Dental Science, School of Dentistry, University of Liverpool, Liverpool, UK.

Dr J. D. B. Featherstone, PhD, BSc, Chairman and Senior Scientist, Eastman Dental Center, Rochester, New York, USA. (Role of saliva in demineralisation and remineralisation of teeth.)

Dr Norman Fleming, Professor, Department of Oral Biology, University of Manitoba, Winnipeg, Manitoba, Canada. (Secretory mechanisms of salivary glands and their manipulation.)

Professor Dorothy A. M. Geddes, PhD, BDS, FDS, MS, Head, Oral Biology Group, Glasgow Dental School, Glasgow, UK. (Effects of saliva on plaque pH.)

Dr D.I. Hay, PhD, Head, Department of Biochemistry, Forsyth Dental Center, Boston, Massachusetts, USA. (The functions of salivary proteins.)

Dr I. Kleinberg, PhD, DDS, DSc, Professor and Chairman, Department of Oral Biology and Pathology, School of Dental Medicine, State University of New York, Stony Brook, New York, USA.

Dr F. Lagerlöf, PhD, DDS, Odont Dr, Head Clinical Research Centre, School of Dentistry, Karolinska Institutet, Huddinge, Sweden. (Salivary clearance and its effect on oral health.)

Dr M. Joost Larsen, Odont Dr, Associate Professor, Department of Oral Anatomy, Dental Pathology and Operative Dentistry, Royal Dental College, Aarhus, Denmark. (Calculus, caries and salivary saturation with calcium phosphates.)

Dr E. Newbrun, PhD, BDS, MS, DMD, Odont Dr (Hon), Professor of Oral Biology and Periodontology, Division of Oral Biology, Department of Stomatology, University of California, San Francisco, California, USA.

Professor D. M. O'Mullane, Head, Department of Preventive and Paediatric Dentistry, Dental School and Hospital, Cork, Eire.

Dr J. S. van der Hoeven, PhD, Institute of Preventive and Community Dentistry, University of Nijmegen, Nijmegen, Holland. (Effects of saliva on plaque microbiology.)

Contents

1

Factors Influencing Salivary Flow Rate and Composition

Unstimulated flow rates vary widely between subjects, and those with low rates do not always have symptoms of dry mouth. The main stimulus to salivation is the sensation of taste (particularly acid) —stimulated saliva is better able (because of changes in its composition) to prevent demineralisation and to favour remineralisation than is unstimulated saliva.

Unstimulated saliva

Unstimulated saliva is usually collected with the patient sitting quietly, with the mouth open to allow the saliva to collect into a beaker or similar receptacle over a given time. Alternatively, the patient can spit out the saliva at regular intervals, while swallowing is inhibited (see below). Several large studies have been done of unstimulated salivary flow rates in healthy individuals (Table 1). The average unstimulated flow rate is 0·3 ml/minute, but the normal range is very large and includes individuals with very low flow rates who do not complain of a dry mouth.

Table 1 Unstimulated salivary flow rate (ml/minute) in healthy individuals

Studies	Type of saliva	Sample number	Mean (ml/minute)	SD[a]
Anderson *et al.*	Whole	100	0·39	(0·21)
Becks and Wainwright (1943)	Whole	661	0·32	(0·23)
Heintze *et al.* (1983)	Whole	629	0·31	(0·22)
Shannon (1967)	Parotid	4589	0·04	(0·03)
Enfors (1962)	SM[b]	54	0·10	(0·08)
Shannon and Frome (1973)	Whole	50	0·32	(0·13)

[a] Note the very high standard deviation (SD) from the mean indicating a very wide range of values covering normality.
[b] SM = Submandibular saliva.

Such a broad normal range makes it difficult to say whether or not a particular individual has an abnormally low flow rate. Unless saliva is almost completely absent, patients can be said to have a dry mouth only on the basis of their subjective symptoms. Patients may complain of a dry mouth even when salivary flow is easily measured. Their complaint may then be due to localised regions of dry mucosa. These are most likely to occur in the anterior palatal region where no major or minor salivary gland secretions enter the mouth.

In a study in dental students of the effect of atropine on salivary flow, subjects were asked to note when the onset of dry mouth symptoms began. On average, the symptoms started when salivary flow had fallen by 40–50% of the normal value—despite wide variation in flow rates. Thus, it appears that it is the change in the amount of saliva, rather than the absolute amount, which is important.

In true xerostomia, it may be impossible to collect any saliva by conventional means. For such subjects, salivary function can be monitored using paper strips, which are applied to the minor mucous glands. The amount of saliva can be estimated using a periotron—an instrument which measures the conductivity of the paper strip (proportional to the amount of fluid) and whose main use is in monitoring gingival crevice fluid.

Whether a particular flow rate is high or low is much less important than whether it has changed adversely in a particular individual. Physicians will often take a patient's blood pressure as a yardstick for future measurements. Dentists, however, do not routinely measure the salivary flow rate. When a patient complains of having a low salivary flow, it is therefore impossible to judge whether or not a genuine reduction in flow has taken place. It would therefore be very advantageous if dentists included measurement of salivary flow as part of their regular examination. Just as there are individuals with very little saliva but without discomfort, so there are others within the normal range who feel that their mouth is drowning in saliva.

Factors affecting unstimulated salivary flow rate

Many factors influence the unstimulated salivary flow rate (Table 2).

Hydration

This is potentially the most important factor. When body water content is reduced by 8%, the salivary flow rate decreases to virtually

Table 2 Factors affecting unstimulated salivary flow rate in healthy subjects

Important factors[a]	Unimportant factors
Degree of hydration	Gender
Body position	Age (above 15 years)
Exposure to light	Body weight
Olfaction	Gland size
Smoking	Psychic effects
Previous stimulation	– thought/sight of food
Circadian rhythms	– appetite
Circannual rhythms	– mental stress
Drugs	Functional stimulation

[a] Most factors listed in the first column should be standardised during saliva collection.

zero. For a man of about 70 kg, comprising about 50 kg of water, 8% dehydration means a loss of 4 litres. In contrast, hyperhydration will increase the salivary flow rate.

Body posture

Flow rate also varies with position. A person when standing or lying will have a higher or lower flow rate respectively than when seated. Flow rate also greatly decreases in the dark, but increases with cigarette smoking or olfactory stimulation.

Biological rhythms

The flow rate of saliva peaks (acrophase) during the afternoon and drops to almost zero during sleep (fig. 1). It is therefore important to standardise the time of day at which saliva is collected.

This circadian rhythm also has important clinical implications for the timing of oral hygiene. For this reason we teach our students that the most important time of day to clean teeth is at night before going to sleep. Lots of plaque and food debris and a greatly reduced salivary flow provide maximum conditions for dental caries.

A study has also shown a circannual rhythm in the flow rate of parotid saliva, with a peak value in the winter. A study carried out in Texas found lower flow rates in the summer, and it was assumed that the effect was due to dehydration. It would be interesting to repeat the experiment in a temperate climate. Whether this finding means people are more susceptible to caries in the summer than in the winter would be very hard to determine because caries is such a long process.

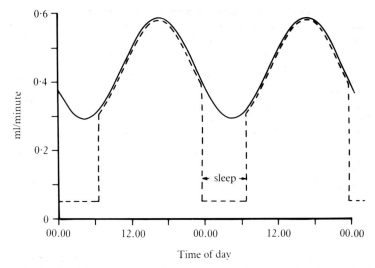

Fig. 1 The circadian rhythm in unstimulated salivary flow rate and the idealised effect of sleep (dashed line) from 2300 hours to 0700 hours (from Dawes, 1972).

Drugs

Many drugs cause reduced salivary flow rate as a side-effect (Table 3).

Stimulated saliva

Several studies of stimulated salivary flow have been done in healthy individuals and show a wide variation between individuals (Table 4). The studies use various stimuli, however, and an international

Table 3 Drugs causing xerostomia

Analgesics (narcotics)	Antineoplastics
Anticonvulsants	Antiparasitics
Antinauseants	Appetite suppressants
Anti-Parkinson's agents	Antiemetics
Antipsychotics	Decongestants
Antidepressants	Diuretics
Antihistamines	Expectorants
Antihypertensives	Monoamine oxidase inhibitors
Antispasmodics	Muscle relaxants
Antiarrhythmics	Sedatives/tranquillisers
Anxiolytics	

Table 4 Stimulated salivary flow rates in man

Authors	Type of saliva	Stimulus	Sample number	Mean (ml/min)	SD
Heintze et al. (1983)	Whole	Paraffin wax	629	1·6	(2·1)
Mason et al. (1975)	Parotid	Lemon juice	169	1·5	(0·8)
Shannon et al. (1974)	Parotid	Grape candy	368	1·01	(0·46)
Ericson et al. (1972)	SM[a]	1% citric acid	28	0·79	(0·38)
Shannon and Frome (1973)	Whole	Chewing gum	200	1·69	(0·57)

[a] SM = Submandibular saliva.

agreement on a particular stimulus would greatly help comparison of different studies.

Factors influencing the stimulated flow rate

Many factors (Table 5) influence the stimulated salivary flow rate, which is, at maximum, about 7 ml/minute for whole saliva.

Mechanical stimulus

The action of chewing, in the absence of any taste, will itself stimulate salivation. Relative to maximum stimulation with citric acid, the flow rate is low, (see Table 4). Mastication also serves to mix the contents of the mouth, thus increasing the distribution of saliva.

Gustatory stimulus

Acid is the most potent of the four basic taste stimuli, the others are salt, bitter and sweet. A study done with various concentrations of

Table 5 Factors affecting the flow of stimulated saliva

Nature of stimulus
Unilateral stimulation
Gland size
Gag reflex

citric acid found that 5% citric acid would stimulate maximum salivary flow rate. The citric acid was continuously infused into the mouth, and the teeth were covered with parafilm to protect them against the acid. For a clinical evaluation, a 3% solution can be placed on the patient's tongue at regular intervals, so that the degree of stimulation is standardised.

Alternatively, for research purposes, sour lemon drops can be used to standardise stimulated flow rate from individual glands. The patient collects saliva into a graduated test-tube in front of a mirror, and with the aid of a stopwatch, the patient can time their saliva flow, and adjust it by changing the intensity of sucking on the lemon drop.

Unilateral stimulus

If a person habitually chews on one side of the mouth, most of the saliva will be produced by the glands on that side, unless gustatory stimulation is also present.

Gland size

Stimulated flow rate is directly related to gland size. This relationship, however, does not apply to unstimulated saliva.

Age

Salivary flow is unrelated to age above 15 years. For a long time it was believed that the salivary flow rate decreased with age. This was mostly because studies had been done on institutionalised, medicated patients. Yet research has shown that aging has little effect on flow rate in normal healthy people. For example, a study of 700 people picked at random on a street in Rochester, New York, looked at stimulated and unstimulated flow rates in people of all ages up to 80 years. The study found stable flow rates across the age span in healthy individuals. The only people with diminished flow rates were those on medication.

Food

Surprisingly, very few studies have been carried out with food as the secretory stimulus.

A recent study tested the effects of seven foods. Even the most bland food (boiled rice) elicited 43% of the maximum flow rate produced by 5% citric acid. Rhubarb pie, which is both acidic and sweet, elicited 70% maximum flow rate.

Further study showed that it was the gustatory stimulus provided by the food, rather than the mechanical stimulus of chewing, which was responsible for these relatively high flow rates. In comparison with other foods, chewing gum elicits a low flow rate (fig. 2). This is because most chewing gums provide a sweet stimulus, which is generally the least effective of the taste stimuli. Initially the flow rate is raised, but as the flavour and sweetness leaches out, only the mechanical stimulus remains, and the flow rate falls. However, gum is chewed for a long time (usually 20–30 minutes) and even this stimulus over a prolonged period can be beneficial, for example in buffering or clearance of carbohydrate.

Unstimulated flow rate and oral health

The unstimulated flow rate is more important than the stimulated flow for general oral health. Unfortunately, there is little that can be done to influence the unstimulated flow rate on a long-term basis, but a recent study has shown that chewing gum (sugar-free) given to students over a long period of time produced a small rise in the unstimulated, but not stimulated, flow rate. This suggests that if we

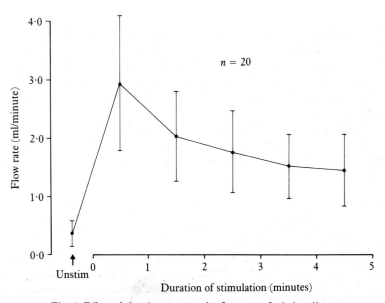

Fig. 2 Effect of chewing gum on the flow rate of whole saliva.

stimulate the glands, even in xerostomia, we may be able to increase their activity.

Carbohydrate clearance from the oral cavity

One major effect of saliva is the clearance of carbohydrate from the mouth. The more rapid the flow, the faster the carbohydrate is cleared. This is true whether the saliva is unstimulated or stimulated, for example by chewing gum. Clearance will be less enhanced if the gum contains sucrose and other fermentable carbohydrates, but if it contains sugar alcohols, such as xylitol or sorbitol, which are minimally metabolised by plaque bacteria, then the increased salivary flow will be very effective in carbohydrate clearance. Recent studies suggest that even sucrose sweetened gum, if it is chewed until the sucrose leaches out, can enhance clearance.

Total daily salivary flow

Studies show that the average unstimulated flow rate over a waking period of 16 hours is about 0·3 ml/minute, or a total of about 300 ml of saliva. During sleep, the maximum flow will fall to 0·1 ml/minute, producing about 40 ml of saliva. The average time spent chewing each day has been estimated as 54 minutes. Studies with various foods suggested an average stimulated flow rate during chewing of 4 ml/minute. So saliva production stimulated by chewing would produce just over 200 ml/day.

Thus the total daily flow of saliva amounts to about 500 ml/24 hours. This is much less than the 1500 ml/24 hours usually quoted in the textbooks.

The composition of saliva

Many factors can affect the composition of saliva (Table 6), such as the type of salivary gland producing the saliva. For example, virtually all amylase in saliva is produced by the parotid salivary glands. Blood group substances, however, derive mainly from the minor mucus glands.

Factors affecting salivary composition
Flow Rate

The main factor affecting the composition of saliva is the salivary flow rate: as the flow rate increases, the concentration of some constituents

Table 6 Factors affecting salivary composition

Species	Hormones
Glandular source	Pregnancy
Flow rate	Genetic polymorphism
Duration of stimulation	Antigenic stimulus
Previous stimulation	Exercise
Biological rhythms	Drugs
Nature of stimulus	Various diseases
Plasma composition (diet)	

rises, for example, protein, chloride, sodium, bicarbonate, while others fall, for example, phosphate, magnesium.

Contribution of different glands

The parotid gland normally contributes 20% of the total volume of unstimulated saliva secretion, while the submandibular gland contributes 65%, the sublingual 7–8%, and the minor mucous glands 7–8%.

At high flow rates, the parotid becomes the dominant gland contributing about 50% to the whole salivary secretion. Since the parotid gland secretes calcium at a lower concentration than the submandibular gland, the calcium content of whole saliva is reduced at high flow rates.

Duration of stimulus

If the salivary flow rate is held constant, then the composition of the saliva depends on the duration of the stimulus. So, saliva collected at a constant flow rate for 2 minutes will have a different composition from saliva collected for 10–15 minutes. The composition will vary depending on whether the gland had been stimulated within the last hour, the time of day, and so on.

Nature of stimulus

This also has an effect on composition, but mainly because of the effect of different stimuli on the rate of flow. However, using constant-flow conditions, the effect of the four basic taste stimuli—salt, acid, bitter, and sweet—on salivary composition was examined. It was found that the type of stimulus used had virtually no effect on electrolyte composition, while the taste of salt stimulated much the highest protein content. There does not seem to be any physiological reason why this should be so. The increase occurred with all protein components—different stimuli did not elicit secretion of different proteins.

Saliva and taste

When saliva is first secreted by the acinar cells of the salivary glands, it resembles a plasma ultrafiltrate. As the saliva passes down the salivary duct, the salivary gland expends a tremendous amount of energy to re-absorb virtually all the sodium chloride and most of the bicarbonate, while secreting potassium. By the time the salivary secretion reaches the opening of the glands into the mouth it is very hypotonic compared with plasma. The osmotic pressure is about one-sixth of that in the acinar cell (fig. 3).

Why does the salivary gland go to so much trouble to produce a hypotonic saliva? The probable reason is to facilitate taste. Taste buds rapidly adapt to the taste of any solution in the mouth including, of course, saliva. Thus, if saliva had the same salt concentration as in plasma (which is very high), we would be unable to taste salt

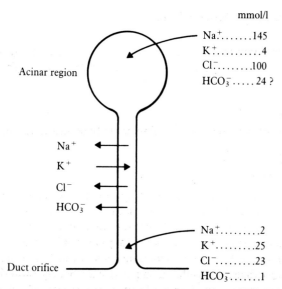

mmol/l

Na^+.......145
K^+.........4
Cl^-........100
HCO_3^-.....24 ?

Acinar region

Na^+
K^+
Cl^-
HCO_3^-

Na^+.........2
K^+.........25
Cl^-.........23
HCO_3^-.......1

Duct orifice

Fig. 3 Changes in some electrolyte concentrations as unstimulated saliva moves down the salivary duct.

concentrations lower than that of plasma. Hence the absorption of sodium and chloride during saliva production, and the resultant hypotonicity of saliva.

Unstimulated saliva is particularly well adapted to facilitate the sensation of taste. Besides being low in sodium chloride (salt), it is also low in glucose (sugar), buffering capacity (acid), and urea (bitter). Recognition thresholds are compared with concentration levels in plasma and in unstimulated saliva in Table 7.

Table 7 Relation of plasma and saliva compositions to taste thresholds

	Salt			Sour	Sweet	Bitter
	Na+ (mM)	Cl− (mM)	H+ (mM)	HCO− (mM)	Glucose (mM)	Urea (mM)
Plasma	145	101	4×10^{-5}	24	4·5	6
Saliva	4	16	4×10^{-4}	3	0·05	5
Recognition threshold	(NaCl)		(HCl)	(NaHCO₃)	(Sucrose)	(Urea)
	12		0·8	10	30	90

The buffering ability of saliva

Proteins

Saliva has a low level of protein compared with plasma, so that too few amino acids are present to have a buffering effect at the usual pH of the oral cavity.

Phosphate ions

As with proteins, there are too few phosphate ions in saliva to act as a buffer.

Bicarbonate

This varies from less than 1 mmol/l in unstimulated saliva to almost 60 mmol/l at high flow rates of saliva. It is the most important buffering system but only at high flow rates, when it is an important buffer against acid produced by dental plaque. However, in unstimulated saliva, the level of bicarbonate ions is too low to be effective. This means that unstimulated saliva is very poorly buffered. It also allows us to taste acid. Any acid put in the mouth will drop the pH and we will sense this as acid.

pH

Salivary pH is dependent on bicarbonate concentration, and an increase in bicarbonate concentration results in an increase in pH. At very low flow rates, the pH can be as low as 5·3, rising to 7·8 at very high flow rates.

Calcium and phosphate concentration

Calcium and phosphate concentrations maintain the saturation of saliva with respect to tooth mineral, and are therefore important in calculus formation and the development of caries (Table 8).

Table 8 Calcium and phosphate concentrations in saliva[a]

	Plasma	Parotid saliva	SM[b] saliva	MMG[c] saliva
Ca (mM)	2·5	0·9	2·0	2·1
Pi (mM)	1·0	3·5	2·9	0·4
Flow rate (ml/minute $^{-1}$) (gland pair $^{-1}$)	–	1·2	1·2	–

[a] From Mandel *et al.*, 1964.
[b] SM = Submandibular.
[c] MMG = Minor mucous glands.

Saliva contains less calcium but more phosphate than does plasma. In addition, as mentioned above, different salivary glands have different concentrations of calcium and phosphate. For example, parotid saliva has less calcium but more phosphate ions than does submandibular saliva, while the minor mucous secretions are very low in phosphate ions.

This situation is somewhat complicated, however, by the fact that calcium and phosphate concentrations greatly depend on the salivary flow rate. Figure 4 shows the effect of flow rate on salivary calcium and phosphate content. With calcium (fig. 4a), the higher the flow rate, the higher the calcium content in both parotid and submandibular saliva. However, the level in submandibular saliva is higher at all flow rates than in parotid saliva. In the case of phosphate (fig. 4b), at all flow rates, the phosphate concentration is always higher in parotid than in submandibular saliva. But while the level of calcium increases with flow rate, the level of phosphate falls.

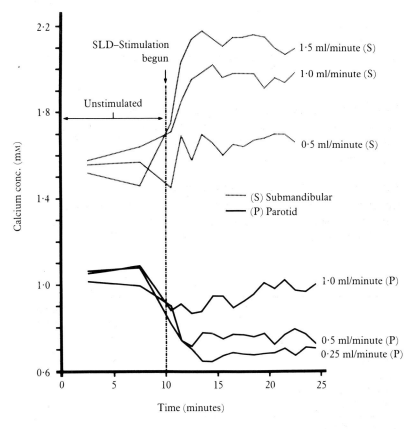

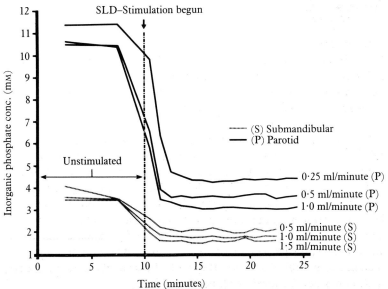

Fig. 4 The effects of flow rate and duration of stimulation on (a) the calcium concentration and (b) the inorganic phosphate concentration in parotid and submandibular saliva.

Theoretically, a decreasing phosphate concentration would seem to be bad for teeth, as it would result in undersaturation of tooth mineral in saliva. But as the flow rate increases, so does the bicarbonate concentration and therefore the pH of saliva. A high pH alters the balance of the different phosphate ions to each other. This results in a fall in $H_2PO_4^-$ and an increase in HPO_4^{2-}, but a dramatic increase in PO_4^{3-}. It is the PO_4^{3-} which is the important ionic species with respect to the solubility of tooth mineral. Thus, although the total level of phosphate falls with increasing flow rate, the important phosphate ion, PO_4^{3-}, actually increases.

If, therefore, we consider the components of the ion product determining the solubility of tooth mineral, all three—calcium ion, phosphate ion, and hydroxyl ion—increase with salivary flow. Thus the higher the flow rate, the more effective is saliva in reducing demineralisation and promoting remineralisation of the teeth. This also means, however, that the higher the flow rate, the greater the potential for calculus formation to occur.

Minor mucous gland secretions

These differ in two major ways from the major gland secretions (submandibular and parotid). First, they are very low in phosphate, and secondly they contain virtually no bicarbonate so they are very poorly buffered. This is quite startling because these secretions are in intimate contact with most of the oral mucosa and hard tissues.

Thickness of saliva film

For too long, oral biologists have generally thought of saliva as a large volume washing over dental plaque. In fact, for most of the time, saliva is a very thin film, perhaps thinner than that of dental plaque. This film, which is about 0·1 mm thick, moves at different rates from 0·8–8·0 mm/minute in different regions of the mouth. This extremely slow speed has implications for the clearance of substances from dental plaque. For example, when plaque is exposed to sugar, acid forms within the plaque. The acid will tend to diffuse out of the plaque along a concentration gradient. But it will tend to accumulate in the outer region of plaque, because it is not being cleared away fast enough by the slowly moving saliva film. This accumulation will inhibit the effect of the concentration gradient and will retard diffusion (fig. 5). This theory might explain the site specificity of caries. Oral regions with a slower moving saliva film might be more

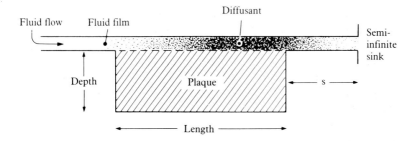

Fig. 5 Diagrammatic representation of the flow of a thin film of saliva over dental plaque and the accumulation of a diffusant (such as organic acid) in the salivary film at the distal edge of the plaque (from Dawes, 1989).

susceptible to caries than regions with a faster moving salivary film because acid is cleared away from plaque more slowly.

Olfactory and psychic stimuli and salivary flow

Generally, olfactory stimuli are very poor at increasing salivary secretion relative to gustatory or mastication stimulation. Similarly, thinking about food or seeing food are also poor stimuli. It may appear that one salivates at the thought of food, but it is more likely that one merely becomes aware of the pool of saliva, always present in the mouth. Although some researchers have measured a small rise in salivary flow with visual stimuli, others have found no effect. In general, therefore, the psychic effect of thinking about or seeing food has little effect on stimulating salivary flow.

Dry mouth—prevalence and aetiology

There have been few epidemiological studies of dry mouth. However, there are about 3 million people in the USA with either primary or secondary Sjögren's syndrome who would be expected to experience salivary hypofunction.

In addition, there are the many people taking drugs which may produce salivary hypofunction as a side-effect. Drug-related hypofunction becomes an increasing problem with age—more people are on medication, often taking several drugs for different conditions (polypharmacy).

One American study of 500 people attending a general practice clinic, found that 30% had dry mouth (< 0·1 ml/minute resting flow).

The patients filled in a questionnaire which asked about symptoms of dry mouth (for example 'do you drink when you are eating?'), and it was found that certain symptoms correlated very well with a salivary flow rate at or below 0·1 ml/minute.

These same symptoms were then studied in the general population. Over 29% of adults (18 000) surveyed at random had symptoms of dry mouth. When asked if they knew what was causing their dry mouth, many of them said it was due to medication. In the same survey, 300 dentists were asked how often they had seen dry mouth. Only one said he had seen it—and then only a single case. This suggests a gap in dentists' awareness, and a failure by dental schools to teach about dry mouth.

In the original study carried out in the general practice clinic many people were found to be on medication. Among those who were not, a significant number were found to be diabetics. Follow-up studies of hyposalivation in diabetics are required to investigate this finding.

Measurement of salivary hypofunction

To diagnose dry mouth it is not sufficient to ask whether or not someone has subjective symptoms. An objective cut-off point of <0·1 ml/minute resting flow is used to define salivary hypofunction.

Measurements should be taken at a standard time of day, because salivary flow varies through the day. The afternoon is preferable, as that is at the acrophase, or peak, of the daily rhythm. But provided the saliva is taken at least an hour after breakfast, there does not seem to be much difference in flow between late morning and the afternoon.

Subjects are asked to swallow, then lower their head, and allow the saliva to drip from the lower lip into a funnel in a graduated centrifuge tube for 5 minutes. Swallowing should be inhibited during this time. At the end of 5 minutes, the subject is asked to spit out whatever is left in the mouth.

A slight variation on this method is to ask the subject to hold their saliva for 2 minutes before spitting it out. This is done three times, so that saliva is collected over 6 minutes in all.

The subjects should sit comfortably with their eyes open, in a quiet room. However, they do not like to be watched, and so must have privacy. They may also be nervous, which may affect their flow rate (either suppressing or elevating it). For this reason, it may be necessary to repeat the measurement a week or so later, after anxiety has been relieved.

Summary—Clinical Highlights

- A patient may claim to have a dry mouth and yet have a significant salivary flow rate.

- Salivary flow rate is nearly zero in sleep. A situation for maximum cariogenic activity will be produced if a person eats carbohydrate and does not brush their teeth before going to sleep.

- Dentists should be aware that many patients are on drugs that have a tendency to reduce salivary flow (for example beta-blockers).

- When salivary flow rate increases, this results in an increase in salivary pH and the bicarbonate content of saliva. These have beneficial effects on plaque pH if the stimulus to salivation does not include excess additional sugar. The increased flow rate will itself tend to remove carbohydrate from the mouth, and will tend to stir up the very thin film of saliva which covers the oral surfaces. The bicarbonate will tend to diffuse into plaque and act as a buffer by neutralising acids present in the plaque, and increase the time for mineral salts to remineralise early caries.

- Saliva is present in the mouth as a very thin film, 0·1 mm in thickness. There is much site-specificity in salivary interactions with plaque, which may have a role to play in the site-specificity of caries.

- Dentists should consider routine measurement of the unstimulated salivary flow rate in patients. This would provide a baseline value for future comparison. A very low salivary flow rate would be an indication of caries susceptibility and would influence the preventive treatment provided by the dentist.

Further reading

Dawes C. Saliva and Dental Caries. *In* G. Nikiforuk (ed.) *Understanding Dental Caries, Etiology and Basic Clinical Aspects.* Volume 1, chapter 9. Basel:Karger, 1984.

Dawes C. Physiological factors affecting salivary flow rate, oral sugar clearance, and the sensation of dry mouth in man. *J Dent Res* 1987; **66:** 648–653.

Mandel I D. The role of saliva in maintaining oral homeostasis. *J Am Dent Assoc* 1989; **119:** 298–304.

2

The Role of Saliva in Demineralisation and Remineralisation of Teeth

Saliva prevents the demineralisation of enamel by its content of calcium, phosphate and fluoride, its buffering agents and its contribution to pellicle formation. Fluoride, even at very low concentration, reduces the rate of demineralisation—these levels may be provided in saliva from fluoride toothpaste, gels, varnishes, and so on. Fluoride also favours remineralisation of enamel lesions, and the mineral which is deposited on the surface of the enamel crystals forms a fluoride-rich, fluorapatite-like coating. Increasing saliva flow may enhance this effect of fluoride.

The caries process

A simplified representation of the caries process is shown in Figure 1. Acid is produced by plaque bacteria when they metabolise fermentable carbohydrate. The acid diffuses through plaque and salivary pellicle and into the enamel where it permeates the liquid phase occupying the spaces between the enamel crystals. It attacks the crystals by dissolving calcium phosphate (demineralisation). The dissolved calcium phosphate must then diffuse out of the tooth before any loss of mineral can be detected. Demineralisation is the loss of mineral from the tooth; subsurface demineralisation is the loss of mineral at a distance below the tooth surface.

Inhibition or reversal of any part of this process will halt demineralisation, and if the conditions are right, result in remineralisation. Remineralisation is the replacement of mineral; this can be partial or complete. Fluoride can enhance this replacement—it speeds up crystal precipitation, and produces a fluorapatite-like coating on the crystals which therefore resist demineralisation more strongly than the original carbonated apatite crystals of the tooth.

Acids and ions move in and out of the tooth by diffusion along

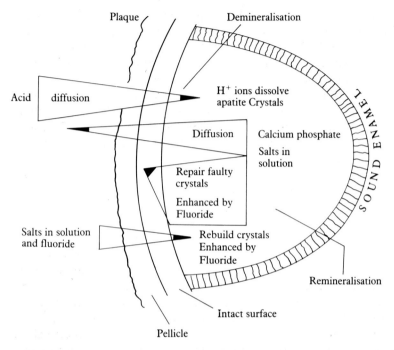

Fig. 1 Diagram of caries lesion formation (reproduced from *Nutrition Today* 1987; May/June : 15).

concentration gradients. Diffusion may be slowed down by the presence of acquired pellicle on the tooth surface.

Acquired enamel pellicle

The acquired enamel pellicle is a selective deposition of salivary proteins and other salivary components on the surface of the tooth. It has been shown to inhibit the loss of tooth mineral (demineralisation), and can be likened to rustproofing on a car. A dramatic demonstration of this was given by a study in which teeth were stored in whole saliva for seven days, while control teeth were left untreated. Artificial lesions were then created in the teeth by exposing them to an acid buffer partially saturated with calcium phosphate. Lesions developed on the control teeth, but no apparent signs of decay could be found on the teeth precoated with saliva. Later work has confirmed this, and suggests that both proteins and lipids from saliva are responsible.

Lipids in general, but especially phospholipids, are highly surface reactive. When there are proteins present as well, a barrier is formed limiting the diffusion of ions. Little is known about how this happens, and exactly what effect this arrangement may have on the rates of movement of ions into or out of the surface is unknown.

The protective effect of the acquired pellicle has been formed to increase as the pellicle 'ages' from 3 to 7 days. Dialysed saliva (lacking minerals and lipid, but retaining its protein content) is still effective in protecting the teeth—albeit less so than whole saliva. The nature of the pellicle changes quite dramatically with time. Not only does it get thicker, but its composition changes as well. Different proteins are added in successive layers.

Enamel, dentine and cementum

Enamel is about 96% mineral by weight or about 85% by volume. Protein and lipid are also present, about 3% by volume, and the remainder is made up of water. Dentine and cementum are quite different in composition to enamel. They contain about 45–50% by volume of mineral, about 30–35% by volume of protein and lipid, and about 20% by volume of water. But all three, enamel, dentine, and cementum, comprise a permeable arrangement of mineral crystals in an organic matrix. The organic material might be thought of as a membrane coating the crystals.

As stated above, for demineralisation to occur, acid must penetrate the organic coating to reach the crystal surface, and then the dissolved mineral must diffuse back out into the saliva. For remineralisation, minerals must first diffuse out of saliva or plaque fluid and through the organic matrix to reach the tooth crystals.

The mineral in enamel, cementum and dentine is a carbonated apatite. It is formed from highly substituted hydroxyapatite in which some calcium is substituted by sodium, zinc, strontium or other cations. About 1 in 6 phosphates are substituted by carbonate, while some hydroxyl groups are replaced by fluoride or to a lesser extent by carbonate. This produces a very reactive mineral compared to pure hydroxyapatite.

Effect of fluoride on the reactivity of carbonated apatite

A series of experiments studied the effect of fluoride on the dissolution of synthetic carbonated apatite in 0·01 M acetate buffer at pH 5 (this is within the range of acid concentrations and pH found within the porous structure of white spot enamel). The rate at which the mineral dissolved was measured, and it was found that adding 1 ppm fluoride to the buffer solution strongly inhibited dissolution of the apatite crystals, whereas incorporating fluoride into the apatite crystal itself made little difference.

Experiments like these have shown that the presence of fluoride in the solution at the crystal surface dramatically inhibits mineral loss from the caries lesion. Relatively low concentrations of fluoride are effective, such as are readily achieved *in vivo* by using fluoride products, such as fluoride toothpastes.

Remineralisation

This term is used to imply not the complete replacement of lost mineral, but simply the regrowth of partially dissolved crystals. This process is also dramatically enhanced by fluoride.

In the absence of fluoride under certain pH conditions, calcium and phosphate will precipitate out of solution to form brushite (dicalcium phosphate dihydrate) $CaHPO_4 2H_2O$. If fluoride is present, however, the fluoride becomes incorporated to form fluoroapatite $(Ca_{10}(PO)_6(F)_2)$. Under the right conditions, precipitation is rapid, and the resultant mineral is one of the most insoluble calcium phosphates found.

Formation of fluorapatite on tooth enamel crystals

A similar process occurs in the tooth when enamel crystals are remineralised in the presence of fluoride, leaving crystals which are coated with fluorapatite. This coating can be detected by magnetic resonance studies or by high-resolution electron microscopy.

A very inactive crystal surface has therefore formed in the place of the original, highly reactive one. The new fluorapatite surface strongly resists acid challenge, and will only dissolve under severely acidic conditions. The crystal surface may thus contain very high concentrations of fluoride (fluorapatite itself contains 39 000 ppm) although the superficial enamel layer only contains about 3000 ppm.

Effect of different fluoride concentrations on demineralisation and remineralisation

The effectiveness of a range of different fluoride solutions from 0–500 ppm, on the inhibition of mineral loss from teeth has been assessed in an experiment in which extracted teeth were exposed alternately to de- and remineralising solutions in a cyclic fashion over 3 weeks, to mimic the intermittent caries attack in the mouth. Daily treatments with fluoride solutions were used to simulate mouthrinsing. A logarithmic relationship was found between the overall mineral loss from the teeth and the fluoride concentration in the daily treatment solution, so that a 50 ppm solution had a marked inhibitory effect, and after a certain concentration, around 500 ppm, there was no further increase in inhibition of mineral loss.

However, with much lower concentrations of fluoride (0·005–0·5 ppm) in the remineralising solution there was a very dramatic inhibition of mineral loss—concentrations as low as 0·04 ppm were effective. These low levels are easily achieved in saliva by the use of fluoride toothpastes, rinses, gels and other topical treatments.

Table 1 shows the range of calcium phosphate and fluoride concentrations found in the stimulated, whole saliva of several hundred people. The calcium level is 0·75–1·75 mmol/l, phosphate 2–5 mmol/l, and fluoride 0·5–5 μmol/l (0·01–0·1 ppm). Very little of the total fluoride found in the mouth is secreted by the salivary glands, about 0·01 ppm. The higher levels of fluoride come from extraneous sources, such as fluoridated water and toothpaste.

Perhaps more important in relation to caries, is the composition of plaque fluid. Plaque fluid is the liquid phase of plaque which is in contact with the tooth. It can be regarded as an intermediate reservoir between saliva and the aqueous environment in the diffusion channels between enamel crystals. Calcium and fluoride concentrations in plaque fluid are similar to those found in whole saliva, while phosphate is approximately double (Table 2). This means that plaque fluid is highly supersaturated with calcium and phosphate ions, with respect to tooth mineral, and that free fluoride ions are also present at about 0·1 ppm.

Table 1 Calcium, phosphate and fluoride levels in human stimulated whole saliva

	Approximate concentration ranges	
	mmol/l	ppm
Calcium	0·75–1·75	30–70
Phosphate	2·0–5·0	60–155
Fluoride	0·0005–0·005	0·01–0·10

Table 2 Calcium, phosphate and fluoride levels in plaque fluid[a]

	Mean (SD) values	
	mmol/l	ppm
Calcium ion	0·85 (0·52)	34 (21)
Phosphate	11·5 (3·3)	356 (102)
Fluoride	0·0049 (0·0027)	0·09 (0·05)

[a] From Carey et al., 1986.

Fluoride clearance from saliva

A few years ago, a study was published in which fluoride clearance in normal and xerostomic subjects following a 0·05% sodium fluoride rinse was investigated.

In the normal subjects, salivary fluoride levels rose to an average level of 60 ppm within the first minute after rinsing, before returning over the next hour to the baseline level. In xerostomic subjects, however, the fluoride level rose more dramatically because salivary clearance was slower, and remained elevated for about 8 hours.

Thus the clinical situation arises in which reduced salivary flow presents a severe caries challenge, but which paradoxically provides magnificent conditions for the retention of fluoride in the mouth.

Further reading

Guggenheim B. (ed.) *Cariology today*. International Congress, Zurich, 1983. Basel: S Karger, 1984; 1–396.

Featherstone J D B. Diffusion phenomena and enamel caries development. *In* Guggenheim B. (ed.) *Cariology today*. International Congress, Zurich, 1983. Basel: S Karger, 1984; 259–68.

Ten Cate J M. The effect of fluoride on enamel de- and remineralization *in vitro* and *in vivo*. *In* Guggenheim B. (ed.) *Cariology today*. International Congress, Zurich, 1983, Basel: S Karger, 1984; 231–6.

Featherstone J D B, O'Reilly M M, Shariati M, Brugler S. Enhancement of remineralisation *in vitro* and *in vivo*. *In* Leach S. (ed.) *Factors relating to demineralisation and remineralisation of the teeth*. Oxford, IRL Press: 1986; 23–34.

Carey C, Gregory T, Rupp W, Tatevossian A, Vogel G L. *In* Leach S. (ed.) *Factors relating to de- and remineralisation of the teeth*. Oxford, IRL Press: 1986; 163–174.

3

Calculus, Caries, and Salivary Saturation with Calcium Phosphates

Supersaturation of saliva with calcium and phosphate ions partly determines the nature of the mineral in calculus, and the rate and pattern of caries lesion development.

Saturation of saliva and dental disease

Although salivary saturation is a crucial factor in caries aetiology, the small differences in salivary composition between individuals are not thought to affect significantly the level of caries in any one mouth. The caries challenge, powerful enough to overpower all local factors, is closely related to the life-style of the subject, including oral hygiene and food habits, and modified by professional dental advice and by social pressures from relatives and friends.

In contrast, the development of dental calculus appears to be unassociated with lifestyle, although age does seem to affect its prevalence. Some people are heavy calculus formers, while others are not, with no convincing reasons why. Unlike caries, calculus formation probably depends on variations in individual biological factors (for example the composition of saliva and gingival pocket fluid) to a much greater extent.

Calcium phosphates

The calcium phosphates that occur biologically are listed in Table 1. Each phosphate will form a separate entity if well crystallised, with their own characteristic crystals, ionic arrangements, and solubility products. But if the calcium phosphate is poorly crystallised, it may be difficult to tell whether the salt will grow into an apatite, an octacalcium phosphate or a β-tricalcium phosphate.

Table 1 Some biological calcium phosphates

Dicalcium phosphate	$CaHPO_4$
Dicalcium phosphate dihydrate (brustrite)	$CaHPO_4 \, 2H_2O$
β-tricalcium phosphate	$Ca_3(PO_4)_2$
Octacalcium phosphate	$Ca_8(HPO_4) \, (PO_4)_4 5H_2O$
Whitlockite	$Ca_{10}(HPO_4) \, (PO_4)_6$
Hydroxyapatite	$Ca_{10}(PO_4)_6 \, (OH)_2$
Fluroapatite	$Ca_{10}(PO_4) \, (F)_2$

Mineral formation

The formation of solid crystals from a solution (such as occurs in calculus formation or enamel remineralisation) occurs by growth of crystals from an initial nucleus. Spontaneous nucleation (or primary precipitation is the spontaneous precipitation of calcium phosphates from highly supersaturated solutions. Some calcium phosphates (for example apatite or octacalcium phosphate) require a high supersaturation before they will precipitate and are often poorly crystallised initially. Other phosphates, such as brushite, will spontaneously nucleate from only a slightly supersaturated solution and always in a well crystallised form.

Heterogeneous nucleation occurs when an extraneous substance, called a matrix or seed, induces the salt to precipitate out from a less supersaturated solution than necessary with spontaneous nucleation. Regular crystals are formed. A seed is a good nucleator if it requires only slight supersaturation to start mineral formation. Pellicle and plaque can act as seeds.

Homogeneous nucleation occurs when nucleation is induced by the presence of a crystal of the same type as that which is being grown. Nucleation of new crystals of apatite does not occur in slightly supersaturated solutions, or in the absence of a suitable seed. However already nucleated crystals may continue to grow at low degrees of supersaturation, as occurs in the remineralisation of incipient (white-spot) caries lesions.

Solubility of calcium phosphates

The solubility of all biological calcium phosphates increases tremendously with a decrease in pH. Thus, when pH decreases, a supersaturated solution may become undersaturated with respect to a particular salt which would therefore dissolve. Conversely, with an increase in pH, an undersaturated solution may become supersaturated to such an extent that the salt precipitates.

This is the reason why salivary (and plaque) pH is fundamental to oral health. A pH decrease may cause mineral dissolution, while on the other hand, a pH increase may cause mineral precipitation.

Composition of enamel and calculus

Dental enamel consists of a fluorohydroxyapatite mixture. It has a fluoride-rich surface, highly substituted with carbonate and sodium. Calculus is formed by precipitation of salivary salts in a matrix formed from protein and bacteria in plaque. X-ray diffraction studies show that calculus can contain: fluorohydroxyapatite, β-tricalcium phosphate, octacalcium phosphate, and brushite. Several different salts may be found in the same sample of calculus, and their relative concentrations vary with the age of the sample. For example, brushite is predominant in freshly developed calculus, and apatite in older, matured calculus. Octacalcium phosphate is predominant in subgingival calculus.

It is not known if the brushite present in young plaque transforms to apatite or octacalcium phosphate with age. At neutral pH, brushite and apatite may co-exist for a long time, and the change of crystal type with maturation of the calculus may be due to an overgrowth of apatite.

The importance of supersaturation in saliva

The concentrations of mineral ions in saliva vary greatly with the source of saliva, degree of stimulation, time of day, and between individuals. Furthermore, the ions in which we are interested can form non-ionic complexes with a number of salivary components. Thus, calcium ions complex with proteins, phosphate and bicarbonate ions. The concentrations of these complexes vary with pH. The saturation of saliva, however, is determined by the concentration of free, uncomplexed ions.

Saliva is invariably supersaturated with respect to both hydroxyapatite and fluorapatite. Indeed, if this were not so, our teeth would spontaneously dissolve and disintegrate. This supersaturation is a prerequisite for the existence of teeth in our mouths. Figure 1 shows the levels of saturation of parotid saliva with respect to the common calcium phosphates at different saliva flow rates.

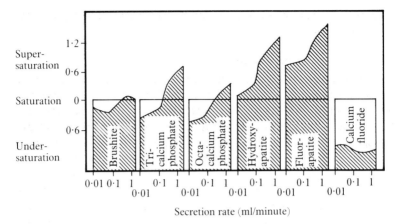

Secretion rate (ml/minute)

Fig. 1 Saturation of parotid saliva with respect to various calcium phosphates often present in the oral cavity: fluor- and hydroxyapatite (tooth mineral and calculus), brushite, tricalcium phosphate and octacalcium phosphate, (calculus) and calcium fluoride (in enamel and dentine after topical fluoride treatment). Within each column the rate of secretion increases to the right. Positive values indicate supersaturation, negative values an undersaturation. (Redrawn from McCann, 1968).

Any apatite crystal in this supersaturated salivary solution will tend to grow. This is why partly demineralised crystals tend to grow or remineralise in white-spot enamel lesions. The same applies to apatite crystals in calculus. In the normal, intact enamel, the crystals are so densely packed that crystal growth is unlikely. However, at a low pH, saliva becomes undersaturated with respect to hydroxyapatite (which therefore dissolves), while still remaining saturated with fluorapatite (which therefore forms). Enamel exposed to such a solution will develop a caries lesion.

Apatite forms a large proportion of supragingival calculus. Octacalcium phosphate and tricalcium phosphate are often present as well. Since parotid saliva is rarely saturated (and then only slightly) with brushite, it is unusual to find brushite in parotid calculus.

The saturation of submandibular saliva is usually much higher than that of parotid saliva. This may explain why calculus forms most readily, close to the submandibular duct orifices. Furthermore, loss of carbon dioxide from submandibular saliva (causing a rise in pH) tends to induce an even higher supersaturation, and a stronger tendency to calculus formation on the lower incisors. This loss of CO_2 has been suggested as a cause of increased calculus deposition in joggers, who mouth-breathe for long periods and thus expose their saliva to the air.

Saliva as a remineralising fluid

There is abundant evidence that caries lesions (whether natural or artificial) can be repaired by remineralisation of partially-demineralised enamel crystals in the mouth and *in vitro*. Saliva is theoretically a less than ideal remineralising solution. It is a poor carrier of calcium phosphates as only 0·003% of the volume of saliva is made up of mineral. If the saliva were not continually replaced, this mineral would be rapidly depleted at the expense of growing apatite crystals, and the supersaturated state would only persist briefly. Nor is it clear to what extent saliva influences the interior of the lesion, where there is intimate contact between the solution in the pores of the lesion and the partly demineralised enamel crystal. The degree of super-saturation in these pores determines whether or not the crystals grow, whether or not there is remineralisation and it is possible that the supersaturation of saliva is too low to survive diffusion through the outermost enamel for crystal growth to occur in subsurface enamel. Thus, remineralisation *in vivo* occurs most easily at the enamel surface, although *in vitro* it is possible to remineralise a lesion completely.

In the mouth, proteins may block the pores in the enamel and restrict the diffusion of mineral ions into the lesions, again preventing complete remineralisation. However, clinically it is not important to remineralise a lesion completely, it is sufficient to arrest it by depositing a non-reactive mineral such as fluorapatite in the surface. Although much research has been done to create a fluid that is a better remineraliser than saliva, so far none has been found—particularly if its fluoride content is optimal. To ensure good remineralisation it is important not to disturb the lesion by probing, as this interferes with the matrix which is to be recalcified. Experimentally, it has been shown that a lesion which has been probed does not completely remineralise, but one which is left alone can remineralise to a large extent.

Formation of the caries lesion

In order to dissolve enamel, a solution in contact with enamel must be unsaturated with respect to enamel apatite. If at the same time the solution is supersaturated with respect to fluorapatite, a caries lesion will develop, because fluoride will be taken up in the surface enamel to form fluoridated apatite, and surface layer will be preserved. A relatively sound surface layer is a main characteristic of the classical white-spot lesion.

The resting pH of the oral cavity is around pH 6–7. Saliva is supersaturated with respect to both apatites at this pH, but as pH drops, the solubility of all apatites increases. Just below a critical value around pH 5·0–5·5, saliva becomes undersaturated with respect to enamel hydroxyapatite, while still saturated with fluorapatite. These conditions favour development of the classical caries lesion.

Soft drinks, fruit juices and other acid beverages are unsaturated with respect to both enamel apatite and fluorapatite. Hence both apatites tend to dissolve out of enamel, giving rise to an erosive-type lesion without any intact surface layer.

Calcium fluoride

Topical application of fluoride causes calcium fluoride to form on the enamel surface. Saliva is unsaturated with respect to calcium fluoride (fig. 1) which explains why this salt is soluble in saliva. A fluoride concentration of about 5–7 ppm would be necessary to saturate saliva with calcium fluoride. Such concentrations are found rarely if at all, and so calcium fluoride dissolves into saliva.

Immediately after a topical fluoride treatment, the amount of calcium fluoride found in enamel is high. But this amount rapidly decreases with time. Figures 2 and 3 show the result of a topical acidified phosphate fluoride solution. Its acidity roughens up the enamel surface and allows deposition of calcium fluoride several micrometers deep into the enamel of the tooth. However, much of the calcium fluoride will dissolve out into the saliva within hours, although a proportion remains for longer; precipitation of phosphate and protein from saliva forms a layer on the calcium fluoride deposit which helps to retain this reservoir of fluoride which is then released slowly into the saliva over days or weeks.

If the same treatment is applied to artificially produced lesions (fig. 4), we find ten times as much calcium fluoride is deposited, and that it is retained for longer within the pores of the lesion. However, eventually, it will dissolve out into saliva.

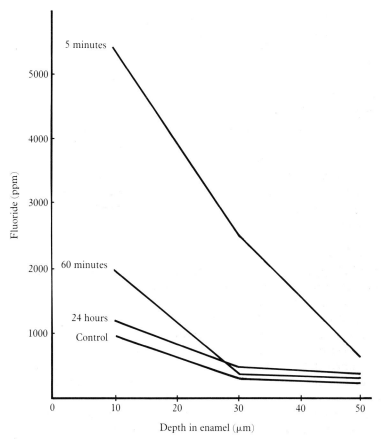

Fig. 2 Amounts of fluorapatite and calcium fluoride at different depths in sound enamel various time periods after a topical acidulated phosphate fluoride treatment plotted as total fluoride concentration. (Redrawn from Brudevold, 1976).

How the cycle of demineralisation and remineralisation can result in more resistant enamel crystals

Once a caries lesion has partially remineralised, that is new mineral growth has occurred on previously present crystals, the new crystal will be stronger and more resistant to demineralisation. In general terms, a new crystal grown on an old crystal seed will usually produce a better crystal.

If remineralisation is taking place in the presence of fluoride, the new crystal formed will be much less soluble in saliva than the old

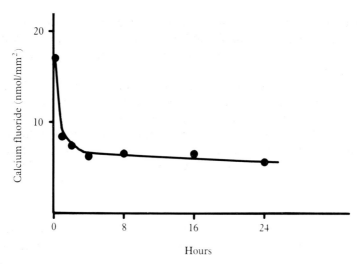

Fig. 3 Amounts of calcium fluoride extractable from the sound intact enamel various time periods after a topical acidulated phosphate fluoride treatment (Redrawn from Larsen *et al.*, 1981).

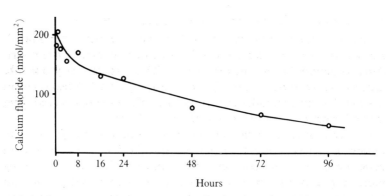

Fig. 4 Amounts of calcium fluoride extractable from an artificial carious lesion various time periods after a topical acidulated phosphate fluoride treatment (Redrawn from Larsen *et al.*, 1981).

crystal. As the cycle of demineralisation/remineralisation continues, the crystal becomes increasingly less soluble and more perfect with time. This occurs in the mouth, and can also be demonstrated in the laboratory.

In addition, there may be proteins, lipids, as well as surface-dissolution inhibitors in the remineralised enamel, which will tend to slow down subsequent demineralisation.

It could be said that a little bit of demineralisation is good for you because it will remove a component of enamel, rich in magnesium and carbonate, and replace it with a fluoride-rich component making the tooth stronger and resistant to subsequent demineralisation.

Remineralising the sub-surface lesion

Some researchers have found it difficult to induce remineralisation in sub-surface lesions because of the relatively sound surface layer that covers the lesion.

However, others have been more successful by reducing the degree of saturation of the mineralising solution. More highly saturated solutions tend to deposit mineral at the outer surface of the lesion. Crystal growth inhibitors (for example statherin from saliva, or methane hydroxydiphosphonate, a synthetic 'crystal poison') can also enhance sub-surface remineralisation by inhibiting crystal precipitation on the surface, thus maintaining pathways for mineral to diffuse into the tooth.

Demineralisation and remineralisation in fissures

Nearly all experimental studies look at what happens to a smooth surface, and yet approximately 80% of lesions, particularly in fluoridated communities, are fissure lesions. These studies may not take access of saliva into account. If, as has been suggested, access is less in fissures than on a smooth surface, then the effects of saliva in reducing lesion formation might be less with fissure lesions.

However, studies carried out on rats whose salivary glands were removed showed a much bigger increase in fissure caries than in caries on smooth surfaces compared with controls. Furthermore, by increasing salivary function in rats, it has been found possible to remineralise caries lesions at the base of the fissures. In humans, caries rarely occurs at the bottom of a fissure but usually halfway up, where the surface is smooth and where salivary access is unrestricted.

Thus it seems that saliva helps to reduce lesion formation in fissures as well as on smooth surfaces.

Acquired enamel pellicle and mucosal pellicle

The acquired enamel pellicle and the so-called mucosal pellicle, are thin films of saliva which coat the hard tissues (teeth) and soft tissues (mucosa), respectively. Both pellicles can be likened to a simple membrane covering the tissues. They are derived from a selective deposition of salivary components, which include lipids, proteins and glycoproteins. The way in which these components are deposited seems to be organised, rather than random, but it is only recently that it has been possible to look at pellicle structure in detail.

In addition to its role as a substrate upon which plaque normally forms, the enamel pellicle may have a role in slowing down demineralisation, and may be important in protecting the teeth against abrasion and attrition. The mucosal pellicle also seems to have a protective action—severe xerostomia results in a great increase in mucosal lesions.

Calculus in children

Children generally have less supragingival calculus than adults, even though they may have a lot of plaque. It is not known why this should be so, although it might be due to different amounts of calcium phosphate precipitation inhibitors in the salivas of children and adults. It might also be due to a different oral flora—conceivably, the organisms may not contain or produce seeds for mineral deposition, or some of the bacteria in children's mouths might produce inhibitors of precipitation.

Further reading

Brudevold F. Fluoride therapy. *In* Bernier J L, Muhler J C (eds) *Improving dental practice through preventive measures.* St Louis; Mosby, 1974.

Larsen M J. Dissolution of enamel. *Scand J Dent Res* 1973; **81:** 518–522.

Larsen M J, Lambrou D, Fejerskov O, Tachos B. A study on accumulation and release of loosely bound fluoride on enamel. *Caries Res* 1981; **15:** 273–277.

Larsen M J, Jensen S J. Solubility studies of the initial formation of calcium orthophosphates and their mutual conversation in aqueous solutions. *Archs Oral Biol* 1986; **31:** 565–572.

Larsen M J, Fejerskov O. Chemical and structural challenges in remineralisation of dental enamel lesions. *Scand J Dent Res* 1989; **97:** 285–296.

Summary—Clinical Highlights

- The arrest and/or reversal of early caries lesions is a natural and very important means of decay prevention which we can enhance by intervention.

- Saliva contains calcium and phosphate in a supersaturated state which reduce the dissolution of tooth mineral in caries, and replace the mineral (that is remineralise the crystals) in early lesions. Salivary dysfunction will essentially eliminate both these functions. Salivary stimulation increases its potential for remineralisation.

- Fluoride in the mouth inhibits demineralisation if it is present in the aqueous phase between the enamel crystals at the time of an acid challenge.

- Fluoride in the mouth enhances remineralisation of early lesions by helping calcium and phosphate, derived primarily from saliva, to regrow the surfaces of partially dissolved crystals. This will produce a fluorapatite-like surface, which is more resistant to subsequent acid attack.

- From a clinical viewpoint, a continual supply of elevated levels of fluoride in the mouth would be a very effective preventative measure.

- The use of methods of delivering fluoride to the mouth (for example fluoridated water, toothpaste, mouth rinses or surgery 'topicals) is a very effective caries preventative measure, even in the case of severely reduced salivary flow. In fact, fluoride use becomes more essential in these patients.

- Because of the supersaturation of saliva, calculus formation would occur much more generally were there no inhibitors of calcification present in saliva and plaque.

Leach S A, Edgar W M. *Demineralisation and remineralisation of the teeth.* Oxford: IRL press, 1983.

McCann H G. Inorganic components of salivary secretions. *In:* Harris RS (ed) *Art and science of dental caries research.* New York: Academic Press, 1968.

Rowles S L. Biophysical studies on dental calculus in relation to periodontal disease. *Dent Pract* 1964;15: 2.

Thylstrup A, Fejerskov O. *Textbook of cariology.* Copenhagen: Munksgaard, 1986.

4

The Functions of Salivary Proteins

Salivary proteins have antibacterial, lubricative, digestive and mineral-binding functions, the latter being important in maintaining super-saturation to prevent calculus formation and enamel demineralisation. Salivary proteins also participate in the formation of the acquired enamel pellicle.

The mouth is a unique, highly complex interface of the body with the external environment. Compared to other orifices, the oral cavity is far more complex, both functionally and biologically (Table 1).

The roles of salivary proteins

Control of the oral microflora

Salivary proteins are important in controlling bacterial and fungal colonisation of the mouth. For example, they modulate the adhesion of micro-organisms to oral surfaces. Various salivary proteins promote the adhesion of particular bacterial species, while aggregating and deleting others. In this way, salivary proteins promote the growth of a benign commensal oral flora.

Other proteins are antibacterial, controlling both the established flora and acting against invading pathogens. For example, sialoperoxidase can control bacterial metabolism, while lysozyme attacks susceptible bacterial cell walls.

Lubrication and hydration

Salivary proteins (for example mucin glycoproteins) also keep the oral tissues moist and lubricated, and help to prevent dehydration of the sensitive oral mucosa.

Mineralisation of the teeth

Tooth mineral is slightly soluble in saliva, and its potential for

Table 1 Salivary protein functions in the oral cavity

Oral functions	Associated problems	Protein functions
Acts as in airway	Air-borne organisms Dehydration	Anti-bacterial systems Water-retaining glycoproteins
Speech	Dehydration	Lubrication system
Taste	—	Gustin
Entry-point for food Mastication Swallowing	Food-borne organisms Soft and hard tissue abrasion	Anti-bacterial systems Lubrication
Control of bacteria, fungi and viruses	Colonisation and infection Controlling pathogens Maintaining commensals Adhesion versus deletion	Anti-bacterial systems Immunoglobulins Glycoproteins Sialoperoxidase Lactoferrin, lysozyme Histatins, others?
Digestion	—	Hydrolysis of starches Amylase
Protection and repair of soft tissues	Toxins, carcinogens Tissue repair	Mucin-rich protective film Growth factors?
Protection and repair of hard tissues Pellicle formation	Enamel mineral is potentially soluble Acid-damaged enamel requires remineralisation	Biologically controlled protective and reparative inorganic environment; statherin, acidic proline- rich and pellicle proteins

dissolving is greatly increased during attack by bacterial acids, and exposure to acidic food and drink. Certain salivary phosphoproteins (for example statherin) inhibit precipitation of calcium phosphate salts from saliva, and so maintain saliva in a state of supersaturation with respect to the calcium phosphate salts which form enamel.

Taste and digestion

Taste has been said to depend on the presence of another salivary protein called gustin which binds zinc. Saliva also has digestive activity, which in man is limited to starch digestion by amylase.

Classes of salivary proteins

In recent years, the number of proteins detected in saliva has increased dramatically. So far, some 40–50 proteins have been detected, but it is likely that more proteins and protective systems will be discovered (Table 1).

Compared to serum proteins, salivary proteins have remarkably varied properties, they range in size from ten-residue polypeptides to multi-million molecular weight mucin complexes. Their isoelectric points span an exceptionally wide range—far wider than serum proteins.

Mucins

Mucins are not like precisely folded, globular serum proteins. In contrast, they are asymmetrical molecules with an open, randomly organised structure, consisting of a polypeptide backbone with carbohydrate side-chains. Their side-chains end in negatively charged groups, such as sialic acids and bound sulphate, which may be important for binding between mucins and bacteria or enamel.

These molecules are hydrophilic and entrain much water. Such structures resist dehydration and are effective in lubricating and maintaining a moist mucosal surface.

Lubricating function

A characteristic feature of asymmetrical molecules like mucins is their reaction to flow or shearing forces. They align themselves along the direction of flow. This increases their lubricating qualities; particularly film strength, which determines how effectively opposed moving surfaces are kept apart.

Aggregation of bacterial cells by mucin

This was the first reported effect of salivary protein on oral bacteria. Interactions between bacterial cell surfaces and mucin-rich films result in the deletion of those bacteria from the mouth.

Bacterial adhesion

Some oligosaccharides in salivary mucin mimic those in the mucosal cell surface. They competitively inhibit the adhesion of bacterial cell to soft tissue surfaces by interacting with reactive groups—adhesins—on bacterial cells, and therefore blocking them. This helps to protect the mucosa from infection. Mucins also interact with hard tissue surfaces, and evidence suggests they may mediate specific bacterial adhesion to the tooth surface.

Secretory immunoglobulins

Secretory immunoglobulins may act similarly to mucins by aggregating bacteria. However, in addition the immunoglobulins are directed at specific bacterial molecules, such as adhesins, or against key enzymes, such as glucosyl-transferase. They may be important in the initial colonisation of the tooth surface and in plaque formation. Although circumstantial evidence exists for complement activity in the gingival crevice, and perhaps in the overlying plaque, it seems unlikely that complement activity could act generally in the oral fluid. Thus, bacterial lysis, which requires complement activity, is not a feature of salivary antibody action.

Lactoferrin

Lactoferrin is present in saliva and has antibacterial activity. Ferric iron (Fe^{3+}) is an essential microbial nutrient. Lactoferrin binds ferric iron, making it unavailable for microbial use. This phenomenon is known as 'nutritional immunity'. A vitamin B_{12}-binding protein has also been discovered, and other salivary proteins may possibly act in a similar way. Some organisms have developed countermeasures to the action of antibacterial protein in body fluids. For example, several *Escherichia coli* strains produce enterochelins. These have higher binding constants for ferric iron than does lactoferrin. Lactoferrin, with or without bound iron, can be degraded by some bacterial proteinases. One spirochete, *Treponema pallidum*, can actually metabolise lactoferrin and use its bound iron for its own nutritional purposes. However, lactoferrin, in its unbound state, also has a direct bactericidal effect on some micro-organisms (for example *Streptococcus mutans*).

Lysozyme

This is one of the best characterised enzymes in the body. It acts on bacterial cell-walls causing cell lysis and death. However, most oral organisms can resist lysozyme attack by developing protective cell capsules or other cell wall variants.

Several oral organisms, including *Streptococcus mutans*, do exhibit sensitivity to lysozyme in assay systems *in vitro*, but it is not clear whether the same are sensitive organisms *in vivo*; access of lysozyme to cell surfaces is unlikely to be so easy, especially when the cells are embedded in plaque.

Lysozyme and other antibacterial systems in saliva presumably keep out susceptible invading pathogens, which are not adapted and do not survive in the mouth. This may be the most important action of the salivary antibacterial system. However, it is very difficult to assess the clinical importance of the different antibacterial systems in saliva, as there are rarely patients deficient in any of these systems. Also, if one group of immunoglobulins is deficient, other antibacterial systems have been found to be elevated; thus the effects of different systems may overlap.

More research is also needed on antibacterial substances when they are adsorbed onto the oral surfaces. Most studies have looked at how antibacterial substances in solution (that is saliva) affect micro-organisms also in solution.

Sialoperoxidase (lactoperoxidase)

Sialoperoxidase acts by catalysing the reaction of bacterial metabolic products with salivary thiocyanate to produce oxidised derivatives (fig. 1). These derivatives are highly toxic to bacterial systems. Bacterial metabolic activity is therefore inhibited by a negative feedback mechanism.

Some micro-organisms have adapted to this control system by

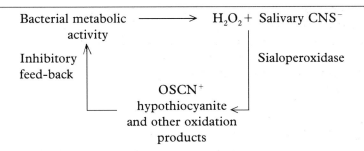

Mediated by sialoperoxidase, bacterially produced hydrogen peroxide and salivary thiocyanate react to give toxic oxidation products. These act by oxidising -SH groups of, for example, glycolytic and carbohydrate transport enzymes. This negative feed-back mechanism significantly inhibits bacterial metabolism, unless organisms adapt, by protecting -SH groups, for example.

Fig. 1 Action of sialoperoxidase.

maintaining unusually high intracellular redox potentials. Further study of bacterial adaptation mechanisms is needed.

Histatins

This group of small histidine-rich proteins, termed histatins, are potent inhibitors of *Candida albicans*. It is not clear how they work, but their discovery suggests possible important functions for other small proteins or peptides present in saliva.

Amylase

Salivary amylase is a calcium metalloenzyme, which hydrolyses the alpha (1–4) bonds of starches, such as amylose and amylopectin. There are five salivary isoenzymes. Maltose is the usual end-product, but if the enzyme is at salivary concentration, about 20% of the end-product will be glucose.

Amylase has a straightforward digestive function, and would also help clean the teeth of carbohydrate debris. But if these are its only functions, why is it also present in other fluids such as tears, serum, bronchial, and male and female urogenital secretions? There have been reports that amylase interacts with some oral bacteria, but again further study is needed.

Enamel—its stabilisation and protection

It is well known that calcium phosphate salts of dental enamel are slightly soluble in saliva. Considering that teeth are exposed to substantial volumes of saliva, far more mineral dissolution into saliva might be expected than actually occurs. The critical factor, however, is the degree of saturation of saliva with respect to the minerals which form tooth enamel. It is well established that saliva is supersaturated with calcium phosphates.

There are obvious reasons why supersaturated saliva is important for teeth. Supersaturation suppresses any tendency for the tooth enamel to dissolve, and under the right conditions, encourages decalcified enamel to recalcify. Supersaturation also occurs in plaque, where it helps protect against demineralisation by plaque bacterial acids.

Theoretically, an inevitable consequence of salivary super-saturation would be the crystallisation of calcium phosphate salts onto the tooth surface. Because this does not normally happen, it was at first assumed that saliva was prevented from being supersaturated by the formation of chemical complexes with the calcium and phosphate ions. However, recent research has now identified in saliva the presence of specific phosphoprotein inhibitors of calcium phosphate precipitation.

Statherin

The first of these inhibitors to be discovered was statherin (from the Greek word σταθεροιοω (statheroiow), to stabilize), a small, highly charged asymmetrical protein (fig. 2). The entire molecule is needed to inhibit primary or spontaneous precipitation of calcium phosphate, but only the first six residues—the amino terminal hexapeptide—are needed to inhibit secondary precipitation (crystal growth). Statherin will inhibit precipitation of DCPD (dicalcium phosphate dihydrate) from a supersaturated solution. It will also greatly delay the transformation of DCPD to more basic calcium phosphates, presumably by inhibiting crystal growth on its surface. Statherin is produced by the acinar cells in the salivary glands. It is difficult to determine the half-life of statherin in the mouth, but it is certainly present in significant concentrations in freshly collected whole saliva to which a protease inhibitor has been added. This would seem to suggest that statherin survives for as long as the saliva remains in the mouth. The half-life of saliva in the mouth is just over 2 minutes, given normal unstimulated conditions.

Statherin is present in sufficient concentration in saliva to maintain a stable and supersaturated environment by itself. But other inhibitory molecules have also been identified. Along with statherin, the main inhibitors of precipitation are the proline-rich proteins (PRPs).

Proline-rich proteins (PRPs)

These are also highly asymmetrical. Almost all crystal growth inhibition by PRPs is due to the first 30 residues at the negatively charged amino-terminal end of the molecule (fig. 3). In fact, the adsorption and inhibitory activity of this segment is more efficient without the positively charged carboxy-terminal part of the molecule. The inhibitory activity of PRPs can be explained by their adsorption onto hydroxyapatite.

Interaction with oral bacteria

The PRP molecule is thought to bind via its amino-terminal segment to the tooth surface. This leaves its carboxy-terminal region directed towards the oral cavity, where it interacts with oral bacteria.

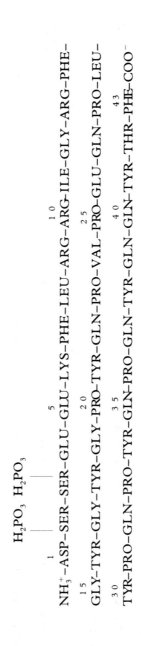

Fig. 2 Primary structure of human salivary statherin.

PO_3^{-2}

PCA – ASP – LEU – ASP – VAL – SER – GLN– GLU – ASP – VAL – PRO – LEU – VAL – ILE – SER – ASP – GLY – GLY –

PO_3^{-2}

ASP – SER – GLU – GLN – PHE– ILE – ASP – GLU – GLU – ARG – GLN – GLY – PRO – PRO – LEU – GLY – GLY – GLN – GLN – SER–

GLN – PRO – SER – ALA –GLY – ASP – GLY – ASN – GLN – ASN – ASP – GLY – PRO – GLN – GLN – GLY – PRO – PRO – GLN – GLN –

GLY – GLY – GLN – GLN – GLY – GLY – PRO – PRO – PRO – GLN – GLY – LYS – PRO – GLN – GLY – PRO – PRO – PRO – GLN –

GLN – GLY – GLY – HIS – PRO – PRO – PRO – PRO – GLN – GLY – ARG – PRO – GLN – GLY – PRO – PRO – GLN – GLN – GLY – GLY –

HIS – PRO – ARG – PRO – PRO – ARG – GLY – ARG – PRO – GLN – GLY – PRO – PRO – GLN – GLY – GLY – HIS – GLN – GLN –

GLY – PRO – PRO – PRO – PRO – PRO – GLY – LYS – PRO – GLN – GLY – PRO – PRO – PRO – GLN – GLY – GLY – ARG – PRO –

GLN – GLY – PRO – PRO – GLN – GLY – GLN – SER – PRO – GLN – COO⁻

Fig. 3 Primary structure of human salivary acidic proline-rich protein–1 (PRP–1).

Studies show that clean apatite surfaces exposed to the oral environment rapidly acquire pellicles of which PRPs are a significant part. More recent work has shown that PRPs adsorbed onto hydroxy-apatite are strong promoters of adhesion of many important oral bacteria. Other research has shown that although several organisms studied had their own profile of salivary proteins to which they adhered, many of the organisms adhered to a single group of proteins—shown to be the PRPs.

This study suggests that PRPs have two functions:
● control of salivary calcium phosphate chemistry
● mediating adhesion of selected bacteria to tooth surfaces.

In healthy mouths, adhesion is a highly selective process. The resultant benign microflora is thus encouraged to colonise the tooth surface to the exclusion of pathogens.

Proline-rich proteins (PRPs) and statherin are present in saliva at birth (or very soon after), that is, before the teeth appear.

Calculus formation and calcium phosphate inhibitors
Calculus formation in plaque occurs despite the inhibitory action of statherin and PRPs. One theory of calculus formation suggests that proteolytic enzymes in plaque interfere with the stabilising effect of statherin by degrading the molecule, including the active hexapeptide segment. Also, calculus formation might be explained by failure of statherin and PRPs to diffuse into the calcifying plaque.

Remineralisation and calcium phosphate inhibitors
Early caries lesions are repaired, despite the presence of statherin and PRPs, because of the relatively sound surface layer of the lesions, which forms an impermeable barrier to diffusion of the inhibitors while being permeable to calcium and phosphate ions.

If either of the inhibitory molecules were to diffuse into partially demineralised enamel lacking a sound surface zone, they might inhibit remineralisation. This effect could be responsible for the many white-spot lesions which never fully remineralise.

However, if the surface enamel is sound, then remineralisation of a subsurface lesion can take place even in the presence of inhibitors on the enamel surface. In fact, inhibitors may encourage remineralisation by keeping the surface pores open and preventing crystal growth on the surface of the lesion. They may thus maintain the pathways through which calcium phosphate ions can diffuse into the tooth enamel.

An additional point is that even though the pores are quite wide during certain stages of the caries attack, it is unlikely that inhibitors will be able to pass through the pores. Even in their degraded but still active forms, they are large molecules compared to pore size. They are also strongly charged, which may also prevent them from entering into the enamel.

No measurements have been done to detect whether or not statherin, for example, can enter the lesion. Only very small amounts would be necessary to inhibit demineralisation, and with present techniques, such a small amount would be very difficult to detect.

Enamel pellicle

The two functions of PRPs are important in the formation of acquired enamel pellicle. This is a 0·1–1·0 μm thick layer of adsorbed salivary protein on the dental enamel surface. It is generally thought to form by the selective adsorption of the hydroxyapatite-reactive salivary proteins, and other proteins associated with them. Bacterial products may also become incorporated into the pellicle.

The pellicle acts as a diffusion barrier, slowing both attack of teeth by bacterial acids and the loss of dissolved calcium and phosphate ions. Although many possible candidates have been proposed, the proteins which contribute to pellicle formation are not well-defined. It seems clear that both mucins and PRPs are involved, but much more research is needed in this area.

Calcium phosphate inhibitors and plaque

The hexapeptide from statherin and the 30-residue amino-terminal segment of PRP might be expected to occur in plaque—acting as calcium phosphate inhibitors. But analysis of large quantities of plaque has found no trace of them. However, plaque bacteria themselves may produce their own calcium phosphate inhibitors. This might be a necessary function to prevent bacterial calcification, which only seems to occur when micro-organisms are dead.

Recently published research has shown that if crystal growth inhibitors are bound to gel particles, and exposed to highly supersaturated solutions, that is immobilised, they can become nucleators of crystal growth rather than inhibitors. A similar situation may occur in plaque, which is very much an immobilised situation, and so encourage calculus formation.

Summary—Clinical Highlights

- An understanding of the protective mechanisms of saliva is extremely important at a fundamental level before there can be effective treatment of salivary problems. This includes the interactions of various protective systems. For example, it has been suggested that the tendency to form calculus could be measured by determining the level of supersaturation of saliva, but this would not take into account other important factors, such as potential bacterial inhibitors of calculus formation found in plaque.

- Synthetic saliva substitutes should, as well as mimicking the lubricating and hydrating functions of saliva, include an anti-bacterial system. More understanding is needed of the possible protective effect of saliva against other harmful agents which can enter the mouth, such as viruses, carcinogens and food toxins.

- If a synthetic saliva is to be made containing calcium phosphate at supersaturated levels in order to protect remaining teeth, crystal growth inhibitors should be included as well. Also, there is now a real possibility of developing proteins which would bind to tooth surfaces and inhibit enamel demineralisation.

5

The Effects of Saliva on Plaque Microbiology

In addition to containing antibacterial activities, organic components in saliva (particularly mucous glycoproteins) support the growth of many oral bacteria; variations in their relative abilities to survive on salivary floral factors can explain some of the variations in plaque microbial composition.

Saliva and the oral microflora are major factors determining oral health. Saliva acts on the microflora by exerting antimicrobial and growth-stimulating effects simultaneously. Little is known about the growth-stimulating (nutritional) aspects of saliva, however, although the various antimicrobial systems have been studied in detail. The role of saliva in supplying nutrients for bacterial growth is the main subject of this chapter.

Antimicrobial factors

The long list of antimicrobial factors in saliva (Table 1) might suggest in fact that there should be no oral bacteria at all! However, these factors are part of the mouth's defence mechanisms against invasion

Table 1 Non-immunoglobulin antimicrobial factors found in saliva

	Salivary glands	Salivary exudate
Salivary peroxidase	+	−
Myeloperoxidase	−	+
Lysozyme	+	−
Lactoferrin	+	+
Aggregating factors	+	−
Histidine-rich proteins	+	−
Amylase	+	−
Anionic proteins	?	?

by pathogenic bacteria, while permitting tolerable levels of commensal organisms which are not normally pathogenic. Many of these factors have been described in detail in Chapter 4.

Factors which aggregate oral bacteria

Salivary aggregating factors are believed to be important and have been well characterised. They act by clumping bacteria together or facilitating their adherence to surfaces. It is not known whether the aggregating ability or adhesiveness of bacteria is related to their abundance in the mouth.

The support of bacterial growth by saliva

Saliva acts as a substrate for bacterial growth. If saliva is sterilised by passing through a 0·2 μm filter and then inoculated with plaque flora or a gingival scraping, a dense bacterial culture will develop within 1–2 days. As in other microbial systems in which there is a mixture of substrates, the carbohydrates are metabolised first and then the proteins; after 24 hours incubation, the carbohydrate level in the saliva culture is low (fig. 1).

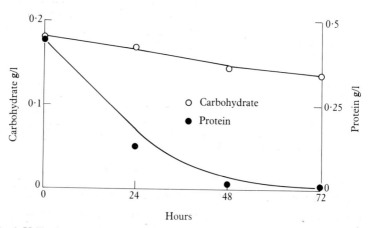

Fig. 1 Utilisation of glycoproteins during growth of plaque micro-organisms in saliva *in vitro*.

Selective growth of bacteria in saliva

Saliva acts as a selective medium for oral organisms. This can be shown by inoculating plaque material into various liquids. If a common broth is inoculated, the final culture will be dominated by staphylococci, while in tapwater it is mainly *Pseudomonas* species. But with saliva, a typical oral microflora develops. Incubations of plaque samples with saliva collected separately from each gland suggest that the composition of the oral microflora which develops depends on the types of salivary glycoproteins present (Table 2). For example one strain of *Streptococcus mitior* prefers to grow on parotid saliva while another strain prefers submandibular/sublingual saliva. Glucose levels in saliva are too low to explain the growth of the plaque.

It is possible that it is the mucin structure which is important in selecting for particular micro-organisms. There is some evidence that gut micro-organisms have adapted to degrade, selectively, particular glycoprotein structures from the intestinal mucus. Similar differences in mucin structure might exist to explain the different types of oral flora in different individuals, but insufficient information is available.

Table 2 Microflora of enrichment cultures showing how different salivas select for different organisms

	Parotid saliva	SM/SL[a] saliva
Streptococcus sanguis	4	8
Streptococcus mitis biotype 1	18	0
Streptococcus mitis biotype 2	0	18
Peptostreptococcus	4	0
Eubacterium lentum	0	24
Bacteroides intermedius	2	6
Bacteroides oralis	40	0

[a] Submandibular/sublingual saliva.

Studies investigating the role of salivary mucins

To study the role of salivary mucins in detail, pig gastric mucin has been used as a substrate, but comparable results have been obtained with human salivary mucin. The pig mucin was made up into a 1% growth medium, containing no other carbohydrate, so that the micro-organisms had only the pig mucin as their carbohydrate source. The growth medium was then inoculated with different oral streptococci, and after incubation the resulting culture analysed for the growth of the inoculated strains.

Interestingly, the various oral streptococci showed different abilities to survive on mucin. *Streptococcus mitior* and other oral streptococci had a much greater ability than *Streptococcus mutans* to use the mucin as a source of carbohydrate (fig. 2). The results also showed that single species were only able to degrade the complex mucin molecules to a limited extent. Utilisation of mucin is enhanced when selected pairs of strains are inoculated together (for example, a strain of *Streptococcus sanguis* and one of *Streptococcus mitior*), suggesting a cooperative action of the two strains.

The different abilities of the various streptococci species to use mucin for growth seems to be related to their ability to produce glycosidase enzymes capable of hydrolysing the oligosaccharide chains. These enzymes are not found to a great extent in mutans streptococci, which is why they are unable to degrade mucin to any significant extent.

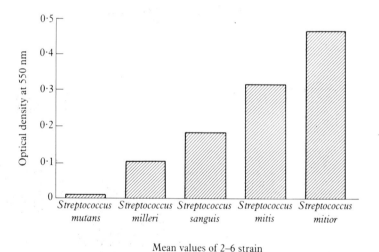

Mean values of 2–6 strain

Fig. 2 Growth of various streptococci in mucin as sole source of carbohydrate.

The lack of ability of *Streptococcus mutans* to use mucin as a source of carbohydrate may be the reason why other, mucin-using species such as *Streptococcus mitior* are relatively dominant in early dental plaque, which is rich in mucins (fig. 3).

Glycosidase enzyme activities are normally determined using arti-

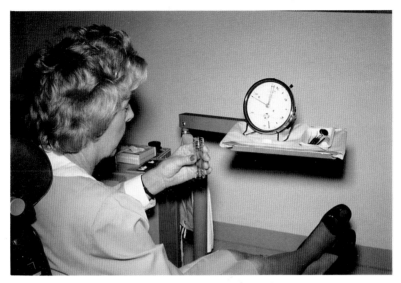

Ready for saliva collection.

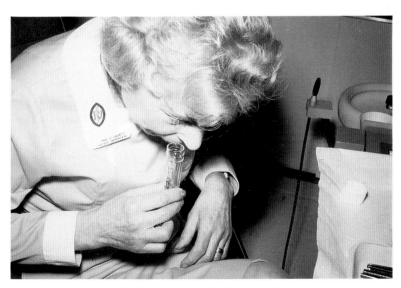

Collecting unstimulated saliva.

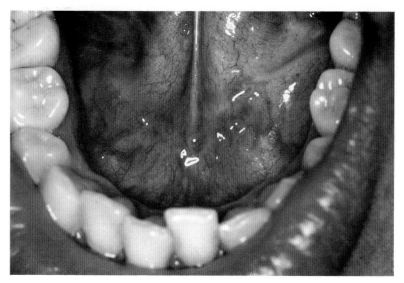

Openings of submandibular and sublingual ducts.

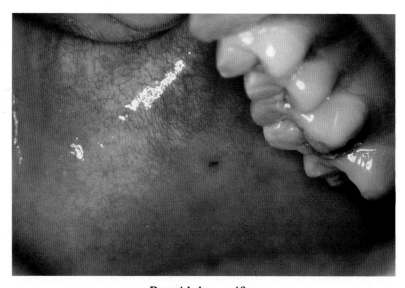

Parotid duct orifice.

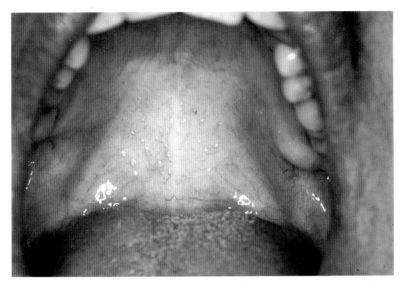

Minor salivary glands of hard palate, showing beads of secretion collecting after several minutes with mouth open.

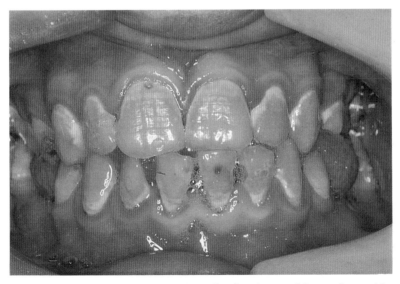

Extensive cervical enamel demineralisation in an older patient with hypofunction of salivary glands.

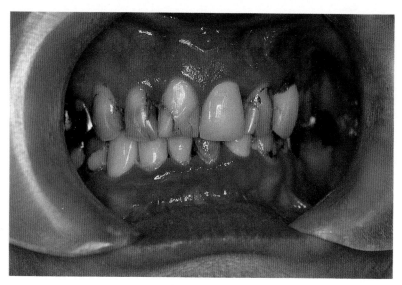

Xerostomia.

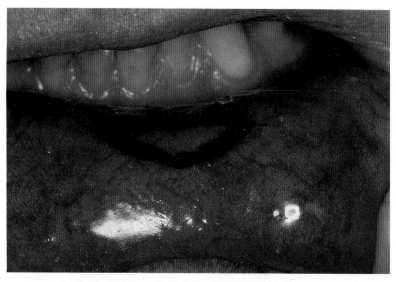

Lower lip marked for minor gland biopsy.

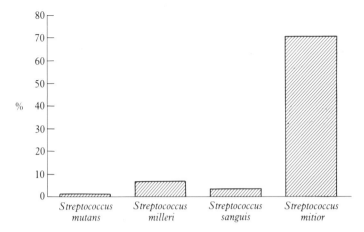

Fig. 3 Proportions of streptococci in early plaque.

ficial substrates. However data from such experiments must be interpreted cautiously with respect to the breakdown of mucin. For example, an organism may not appear to have fucosidase activity against an artificial fucose derivative, but it may still release fucose from the mucin oligosaccharides *in vivo*.

Parallels with in vivo findings

It is interesting to compare the growth of oral streptococci in mucin medium with their occurrence in the mouth. In one study, monkeys were given either water containing sucrose or casein, or plain water to drink. They were also fed by stomach tube, so that no other foodstuffs entered the mouth. When the dental plaque was later sampled, *Streptococcus mutans* was predominant in those monkeys given water containing sucrose, while *Streptococcus mitior* was predominant in those given just water. *Streptococcus sanguis*, however, was predominant in monkeys given water containing casein (Table 3).

These results can be explained by known properties of the three organisms, and show that the type of energy sources available for growth are very important in determining the microbial composition of plaque. Micro-organisms can be grouped according to their preferred substrate. The results also parallel the earlier findings in culture media that streptococcal species grow on mucin, but that *Streptococcus mitior* grows better than *Streptococcus mutans* when mucin is the only source of nutrients.

Table 3 Streptococcal species in early dental plaque in tube-fed monkeys as a percentage of total microflora[a]

	Sucrose	Casein	Water
Streptococcus mutans	50%	0%	0%
Streptococcus sanguis	7%	48%	21%
Streptococcus mitior	4%	9%	34%
Streptococcus salivarius	2%	4%	1%

[a] From Kilian and Rölla, 1976.

Thus, saliva alone selects for a non-cariogenic microflora with low levels of *Streptococcus mutans*. In passing, note should be taken when developing saliva substitutes that substrates are not added which would stimulate the numbers of mutans streptococci.

In the mouth, salivary glycoproteins are also found either as a mucosal film, or on the teeth, as the acquired pellicle. The pellicle will differ in composition from ductal saliva, as only certain components of saliva actually bind to the mucosa or tooth surface. Binding of bacteria to the acquired pellicle must also be taken into account in the selection of the flora.

Summary—Clinical Highlights

- In general, bacteria can proliferate and live in the mouth. Saliva has a protective function in regulating the oral microflora, not only in keeping pathogens out, but also in maintaining the natural microflora. Saliva also acts as a source of nutrients for bacterial micro-organisms.

6

Effects of Saliva on Plaque pH

Saliva can exert major effects on the pH of plaque, partially independent of the metabolism of carbohydrates. The pH response to foods is a function both of salivary effects and of plaque acid production. Saliva can provide substrates for base production, especially marked in subjects with kidney disease.

Acidogenic bacteria in dental plaque can rapidly metabolise certain carbohydrates to acid end-products. In the mouth, the resultant change in plaque pH over time is called a Stephan curve. It has a characteristic shape, the pH decreases rapidly at first to a minimum pH before increasing again gradually (fig. 1).

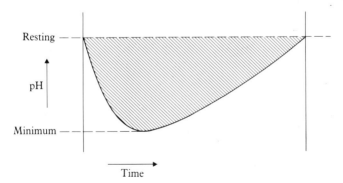

Fig. 1 Diagram of the Stephan curve—the plaque pH response to ingestion of fermentable carbohydrate. (Reproduced from Rugg-Gunn *et al.*, *Br Dent J* 1975; **139:** 351–356.)

Factors affecting the Stephan curve

Various interacting factors can influence the shape of a Stephan curve, and it is extraordinarily difficult to assess the relative contributions of different factors, although a start has been made using simulated computer models.

The decrease in pH

Two main factors affect the rate at which the pH decreases:
- the presence of exogenous, rapidly fermentable carbohydrate, usually sugars
- low buffering capacity of saliva at resting salivary flow rates.

The minimum value of pH

The minimum value of pH and how long the pH stays at that minimum is determined by several factors:
- whether any fermentable carbohydrate remains in the mouth, and whether the carbohydrate has been cleared for example, by swallowing, rather than being metabolised by bacteria
- the pH may fall to values at which bacterial enzyme systems cease to function properly
- the buffering capacity, both in plaque and saliva, but particularly in stimulated saliva, may be critical.

The steady rise in pH is influenced by all the factors mentioned above, including diffusion of acids out of the plaque into saliva. It is also affected by the production of bases in the plaque itself, which act to bring the plaque pH back up towards a more neutral level, and by active removal of acids: for example, by further metabolism of lactate by species of Veillonella to less acidic products. Some of the acetate and lactate will also be lost by diffusion into enamel. The breakdown of carbohydrates stored by bacteria within plaque may also slow the pH rise.

The importance of saliva in restoring plaque pH

Some 30 years ago, researchers compared the Stephan curves produced following a sucrose rinse, with and without salivary restriction. The results showed that excluding saliva by cannulating the ducts of the major glands and diverting the saliva outside the mouth, lowered the minimum pH and slowed recovery to the baseline pH (fig. 2).

Increase in lactate as pH decreases

An experiment done many years ago proved that the fall in plaque pH was associated with an increase in lactate levels. Initially, under resting conditions, relatively high concentrations of acetate and propionate compared to lactate were found in the plaque. However once the plaque had been exposed to fermentable sugar, by eating a sugar lump, lactate production increased dramatically. Simulta-

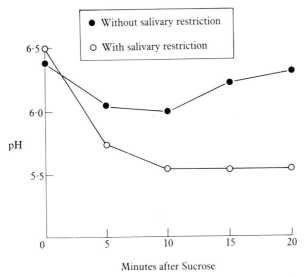

Fig. 2 The effect of restricting the access of saliva to plaque upon the shape of the Stephan curve. (Reproduced from Jenkins, *Physiology of the Mouth*. London: Blackwell, 1978.)

neously, acetate and propionate were lost from the plaque. At the time, these acids were thought to be lost to saliva, but later work has indicated that some of them may diffuse from the plaque into the tooth. The nature of the acids in plaque may be important because they differ in their ability to attack the enamel.

Within the next 30 minutes, the pH had almost returned to its resting level. However the acid anion profile (the proportion of different acid anions such as lactate and acetate in plaque) did not return to resting levels until much later. The presence of relatively high acetate concentrations in resting plaque is due to the accumulation of end-products of amino acid breakdown as well as those of carbohydrate catabolism.

Serial eating of sugar compared to one-off consumption

On one occasion, subjects were asked to chew one sugar lump, and then on another occasion to eat five sugar lumps in a row. When just one sugar lump was eaten, the Stephan curve dropped and then recovered quickly to the resting pH. However, the Stephan curve fell to a lower minimum pH and took longer to recover when five sugar

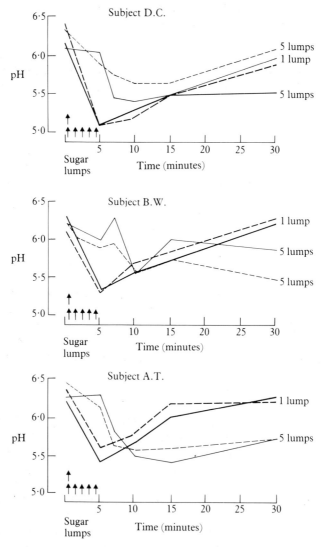

Fig. 3 Stephan curves in three individuals following consumption of one or five sugar lumps in succession. (Reproduced from Geddes, *Caries Res* 1975; **9**: 98–109.)

lumps were chain-chewed. This showed there had been a change in the plaque pH response, brought about by prolonged acid production (fig. 3).

However, it is also interesting to note that plaque pH didn't really begin to drop dramatically until after mastication had finished, and the effect of five lumps eaten together is less than the cumulative effect of five separate lumps spaced apart.

Other carbohydrates

Most experiments on plaque pH have been done with sucrose or glucose, but there have been studies on other types of carbohydrates, such as other mono- and disaccharides, and on starch. Further study is needed on the fate of these carbohydrates in the oral cavity, their rate of clearance, duration of retention, and their effect on plaque pH, as the present evidence is incomplete or inconsistent.

Polysaccharide production

Many oral micro-organisms produce extracellular polysaccharides in the presence of excess sucrose. These include glucans which are thought to increase plaque adhesion and thickness, as well as other polysaccharides which are subsequently broken down to acid. Some micro-organisms build up intracellular polysaccharide stores, the breakdown of which is an ongoing contribution to acid production.

Age and site of plaque

These are important mainly in so far as they influence the microbial composition and thickness of plaque and the access of saliva. The age of plaque is usually defined as the time elapsed since plaque was last removed, for example, by scaling or very thorough home toothcleaning. But this definition is limited because plaque is always being disturbed and removed by the action of the tongue and cheeks and by foods. The thickness of plaque, therefore, is probably more important. Thickness affects microbial composition and how easily substances can diffuse through plaque. Thicker plaques are more anaerobic, and so in the inner layers will favour the growth of strictly anaerobic species. The rate of penetration of nutrients will depend on the cube of the thickness of the plaque, and also on whether the nutrient molecule has negative or positive charged groups. Calcium and phosphate levels in plaque increase with time, 10-day-old plaque has about 25% of the mineral content of calculus.

Buffering systems of plaque

A large range of plaque pH values seems to be compatible with oral health, and as with salivary flow rates, what may be healthy for one individual may be unhealthy for another. This is due to the multifactorial nature of dental caries.

Buffering systems

Plaque has an intrinsic buffering capacity, due to the presence of phosphates and bicarbonates, and to proteins and other macromolecules in plaque. Saliva, however, also contributes several buffering systems, including bicarbonate, phosphates and proteins.

Calcium phosphate crystals are thought to be present even in young plaque and can dissolve under acid conditions to increase greatly the buffering capacity. This can also raise the concentrations of calcium and phosphate ions, and thus help to oppose the demineralisation of the tooth. A negative correlation exists between calcium phosphates in plaque, and caries activity.

Bicarbonate

Metabolically derived bicarbonate increases with salivary gland activity, so that bicarbonate provides an increasingly effective buffer system against acid, especially at high flow rates. Salivary pH also rises with the increase flow rate, so in addition to its buffering effect, stimulated saliva neutralises plaque acidity.

Base formation

Saliva has detectable levels of ammonia, a base that neutralises acid, and also of urea. Certain members of the oral flora can convert urea in saliva and plaque to ammonia. In addition, some bacteria can decarboxylate the amino acids from salivary peptides to form amines— these are alkaline and also remove hydrogen ions from the system. Arginine and lysine-containing peptides are especially effective substrates for amine production.

Metabolic state of plaque and pH value

If plaque is 'starved', that is no fermentable carbohydrate is eaten for 8–12 hours, plaque pH is normally between 7–8. Lactate is usually absent, and relatively high levels of acetate and propionate are found. The term 'resting plaque' normally refers to plaque 2–2·5 hours after the last intake of exogenous carbohydrate. At this point the pH is usually between 6 and 7. The acid anion profile includes a low level of lactate, and some acetate and propionate.

The dietary history of plaque is one of the most important factors affecting the Stephan curve. Even a modest restriction of sugar intake for 1–2 days will considerably influence the shape of the curve. For example, when plaque pH in humans is compared before and after a sequence of sucrose rinses over 3 weeks, there will be a decrease in both the resting pH and the minimum pH.

An increase in lactate favours growth of veillonella species, so the presence of this organism is an indication of homofermentative pathways—the more lactic acid produced, the more veillonella.

Enhanced salivary stimulation and its pH-raising effects

The effect of chewing a sugarless gum and a sugar-containing gum have been compared. Chewing a sugarless gum produced a rise in plaque pH, reflecting the raised pH of stimulated saliva. But with a sugar-containing gum, despite a stimulated salivary flow, there was a decrease in pH which lasted for 20 minutes (fig. 4). Chewing would therefore seem to have a beneficial effect on plaque pH by promoting salivary flow, but this effect may be reduced by the presence of fermentable carbohydrates. However, recent work suggests that if sugarless or sugar-containing gum is chewed after the plaque is

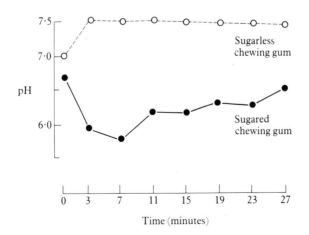

Fig. 4 Plaque pH responses to chewing sugarless or sugared chewing gum. (Reproduced from Rugg-Gunn *et al.*, *Br Dent J* 1978; **145**: 95–100.)

acidified by eating fermentable carbohydrate, both have a beneficial effect on neutralising plaque pH; the duration and time of chewing are critical. This suggests that the additional substrate for acid production provided by the sugared gum is less of a factor.

Chewing even an unflavoured, unsweetened material like paraffin wax has a striking effect on plaque pH. Very shortly after chewing, the pH rises. This effect is not due so much to the cessation of acid production, but to the increased bicarbonate buffering that occurs with an increased salivary flow rate. The level of bicarbonate in saliva in response to chewing gum can reach 12–13 mmol/l, and it is remarkable how quickly this can elevate pH.

However, salivary pH can show a pH fall as well. For example, although stimulated saliva can raise the pH, in some studies, consumption of carbohydrates can lead to the production of enough acid from the tongue microflora to decrease salivary pH as low as pH 5. This will reduce the protective buffering of plaque by saliva.

In another experiment, plaque pH was measured following a sequence of chewing—a sugar-free gum, followed by a piece of paraffin wax, and finally a sucrose rinse. The change in plaque pH over time elicited by the sucrose rinse followed a typical Stephan

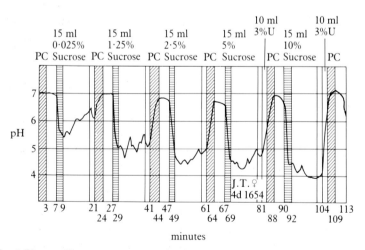

Fig. 5 Plaque pH measurements recorded from a pH electrode mounted interdentally in a partial denture, after rinsing with increasing concentrations of sucrose solutions (PC = chewing paraffin wax; U = urea 3% mouthrinse). (Reproduced from Imfeldt, *Schweiz Monats Zahan* 1977; **87:** 448.)

curve. This suggests that, in this case at least, there was no carry-over effect from chewing to prevent subsequent acid production.

Some studies of plaque pH use the technique of chewing paraffin wax or using a urea rinse to bring the plaque pH back to normal after a carbohydrate challenge. Figure 5 shows the effect of a range (0·025–10%) of sucrose concentrations on plaque pH. At a low sucrose concentration, there was a small decrease in plaque pH which returned to resting values quite quickly, even without the aid of a paraffin chew. However, at higher sucrose concentrations, the pH value did not return to pH 7, even after a 5% urea rinse, before the next sucrose challenge. This indicates that there was ongoing sugar metabolism in the plaque. These results show that simple measurement of pH does not necessarily indicate the metabolic processes going on in the plaque; just because a pH value is 7, does not mean that carbohydrate breakdown is not occurring in the plaque. This implies that pH should be measured for an extended period of time. Measurement of the concentrations of the acid products of metabolism gives a more direct indication of plaque activity in the mouth.

Caries-resistant versus caries-susceptible people

It has been known since the 1940s that people with minimal caries tend to have a high Stephan curve (low plaque acidity), while people with a lot of decay have a low Stephan curve (high plaque acidity). Some recent studies of subjects who are caries-free despite consuming a potentially cariogenic diet have shown that these individuals do not exhibit a normal Stephan curve in response to sucrose exposure. Early indications suggest that their plaque has a highly active base-forming metabolism.

When a sucrose stimulus is given in the form of chewing gum, there is a decrease in plaque pH in both groups, but the decrease is greater in the caries-susceptible subjects. If saliva is then excluded, the resulting drop in pH is much more rapid in the caries-susceptible subjects (fig. 6).

Salivary clearance and plaque pH

It is interesting to speculate whether caries-resistant subjects have faster rates of clearance of fermentable carbohydrate than those who are caries-susceptible. People with rapid clearance rates have a shallow Stephan curve, while those who clear more slowly have deeper curves. Some preliminary studies have suggested that the

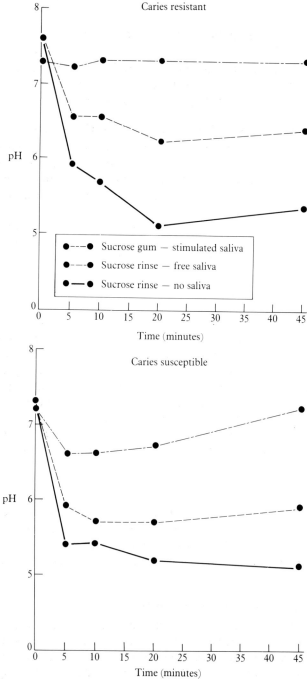

Fig. 6 Stephan curves from caries-resistant and caries-susceptible subjects, after a sucrose challenge under different conditions of salivary access. (Reproduced from Abelson and Mandel, *J Dent Res* 1981; **60:** 1636.)

residual volume of saliva after swallowing is related to caries experience. The residual volume is important in determining the clearance
rate—the smaller the volume, the faster the clearance.

Clearance rates in different regions and plaque pH

Studies have shown that the labial and upper anterior region is a site
of slow clearance, the lingual and lower anterior region is a site of
rapid clearance, and the buccal area a site of intermediate clearance.
Further work is required to map the pattern of clearance in other
regions of the mouth.

The plaque pH in these regions relates well to the rate of clearance.
The approximal surfaces of the upper anteriors have the lowest
plaque pH, since clearance is slower from these sites. This also relates
to the caries prevalence in anterior teeth, being higher in upper than
lower approximal surfaces.

Saliva as a transport mechanism within the mouth

If plaque pH is measured simultaneously on both sides of a subject's
mouth, and the subject sucks a sweet on one side of the mouth, then
pH change on the 'sweet' side shows a very rapid drop in pH, but
there is a delay before the pH drops on the other side, and it does not
fall as low. Presumably the saliva does not equally distribute the
carbohydrate round to the other side of the mouth.

In addition to transport of carbohydrate substrate, saliva also
distributes fluoride and other preventive agents unequally to different
parts of the mouth.

Antibacterial factors

Antibacterial factors are thought to stabilise the microbial flora within
the oral cavity. The contribution of antimicrobial factors to the effect
of saliva on the Stephan curve is poorly defined. However, the
lactoperoxidase/thiocyanate system can reduce the acidogenicity of
plaque.

Plaque pH in renal dialysis children

Children on renal dialysis have high concentrations of ammonia and
urea in saliva compared with normal children. In one study we found
that although the children on dialysis ate many sweets often, they had
a lower caries experience than did the control children. It is likely that
this is due to a direct effect of salivary ammonia and urea on plaque

pH, as the plaque from these children was shown to be capable of forming acid from sugars.

Fluoride levels and plaque pH

Salivary fluoride levels, even in a fluoridated area and after using fluoride toothpaste, are quite low, about 1 μmol/l.

It has been shown that an increased systemic intake of fluoride will lead to an elevated level of plasma fluoride and subsequently raised salivary levels. This can lead to increases in plaque fluoride level. We also know that a high level of fluoride is retained in plaque for up to 8 hours after a fluoride rinse.

The extent to which systemic fluoride administration can affect bacterial activity in the plaque is not known, but plaque fluoride levels are usually 50–100 times higher than that in whole saliva. Topically administered fluorides have antibacterial actions, but this is a direct effect and not mediated by saliva. However, fluoride from dentifrices, gels and other vehicles may precipitate on the tooth surface as calcium fluoride, which then slowly dissolves into the saliva and elevates the salivary fluoride concentration slightly.

Systemic fluorides have only a small effect on plaque acid production, but their effect may be great enough to tip the scales between demineralisation and remineralisation of tooth enamel. Part of the fluoride in plaque is present in a bound form, but part is released into solution when the pH falls. This can also be potentially beneficial in favouring remineralisation and modifying subsequent bacterial metabolism.

Further reading

Edgar W M. The role of saliva in the control of pH changes in human dental plaque. *Caries Res* 1976; **10:** 241–254.

Edgar W M. Duration of response and stimulus sequence in the interpretation of plaque pH data. *J Dent Res* 1982; **61:** 1126–1129.

Geddes D A M. The production of L(+) and D(-) lactic acid and volatile acids by human dental plaque and the effect of plaque buffering and acidic strength on pH. *Archs Oral Biol* 1972; **17:** 537–545.

Geddes D A M. Acids produced by human dental plaque metabolism *in situ*. *Caries Res* 1975; **9:** 98–109.

Lindfors B and Lagerlöf F. The effect of sucrose concentration in saliva after a sucrose rinse on the hydronium ion concentration in dental plaque. *Caries Res* 1988; **22:** 7–10.

Mandel I D. Impact of saliva on dental caries. *Compend Contin Educ Dent Suppl* 1989; **13:** S476–481.

Summary—Clinical Highlights

- Saliva is essential to the balance of plaque acid and base. pH is a measure of the acid-base balance; however, pH alone may not reflect accurately the metabolic activities in plaque. Raising plaque pH while retaining rapidly fermentable carbohydrate in plaque may not remove the potential for future acid production. Finally, the salivary factors affecting plaque pH (and thus caries) can vary from site to site in the mouth.

7

Salivary Clearance and its Effect on Oral Health

Mechanisms of salivary clearance of carbohydrates from food, acids from plaque, and therapeutic substances (for example fluoride) help to explain differences in oral health between different individuals, and between different sites within a single mouth.

A large number of substances of different chemical composition pass through the oral cavity every day. Some of these substances, such as sucrose or acids, are a threat to the health of the oral cavity with its unique and vulnerable tissues. Other substances, like fluoride or chlorhexidine, act as a defence, promoting oral health.

Many substances will dissolve into saliva from which they will then diffuse out into the oral tissues. The effect of incoming freshly secreted saliva, however, is to dilute the concentration of dissolved substances, a process that is described as salivary clearance.

Thus, a rapid salivary clearance of harmful substances would be beneficial for oral health, while the reverse would be true of protective substances.

Models for salivary clearance
Swenander-Lanke model
The first model for salivary clearance was suggested by Swenander-Lanke in the mid-1940s. Her model was very simple. A chemical—sucrose—enters the oral cavity at a certain concentration and saliva flows at a constant rate into the mouth, and is removed (swallowed) at the same rate (fig. 1). In experimental studies, plotting the logarithm of the concentration of sucrose versus time resulted in a straight line. The decrease in concentration can also be described by using the 'halving time', that is the time it takes for the sucrose to decrease in concentration by half. Alternatively, one can measure the time it takes for the concentration of the substance to reach a given low level.

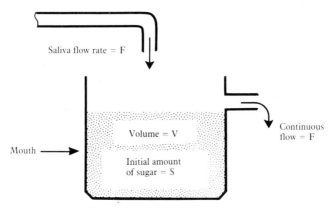

Fig. 1 Model for oral clearance as suggested by Swenander-Lanke (1957). Saliva is swallowed at the same rate as produced by the salivary glands.

Oral cavity as an incomplete siphon

A more recent model by Dawes describes the oral cavity as an incomplete siphon (fig. 2). According to this model, after swallowing there is a minimum level of saliva remaining in the mouth, called the residual volume of saliva. Saliva then flows into the mouth at a rate dependent on the stimulating effect of an ingested substance. The volume of saliva in the mouth increases until a maximum volume is reached. This stimulates the subject to swallow, clearing some of the

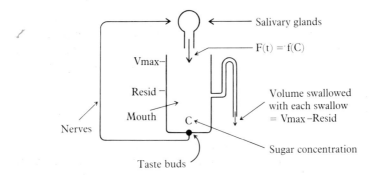

Fig. 2 Amended model for oral clearance suggested by Dawes (1983). Saliva is produced in a rate dependent on the concentration of sugar in the saliva. When a maximum volume of saliva (VMAX) is reached a swallow occurs and the salivary volume decreases to a residual volume (RESID) eliminating some of the sugar.

substance to be eliminated from the oral cavity. The remainder (dissolved in the residual volume of saliva) is then progressively diluted by the saliva again entering the mouth until the maximum volume is reached, and another swallow occurs. Other studies have indicated that clearance occurs in two stages, rapidly from the bulk of the saliva, and more slowly from stagnation areas (for example between the teeth). Studies of clearance in edentulous people would be of interest to test this two-compartment concept.

The Dawes model has been used to describe with considerable accuracy the clearance of substances such as sucrose.

Fluoride clearance

In the case of fluoride, which is also present in the saliva entering the mouth, and which reacts with the teeth and with plaque, the model requires further refinement. For example, plaque fluoride levels can be elevated for 6–8 hours following a rinse and can constitute a 'reservoir' of fluoride.

During the early phase of clearance, some of the fluoride, for example, will diffuse into the plaque from which it is later redistributed into the bulk saliva compartment. This will delay clearance of fluoride, as will the formation of calcium fluoride deposits on the teeth which can occur at higher fluoride concentrations and alter the clearance pattern.

Some fluoride may be swallowed, absorbed into the blood and then partly recycled via the salivary glands. Some clearance curves for fluoride show an initial fall followed by a rise, suggesting recycling via saliva. If all of these factors are built into a computer model, it is possible to evaluate the effects of a single variable while keeping other variables constant. The variables I will discuss here are: the residual and maximum volumes, and the unstimulated and stimulated flow rates.

Volume of saliva in the mouth after swallowing (residual volume)

The average residual volume is approximately 0·8 ml, but the range is very large, suggesting that residual volume may be important in individual differences in clearance patterns. Using the computer model, the effect of varying the residual volume on clearance curves was very large (fig. 3).

In fact, the difference between the clearance curves obtained with

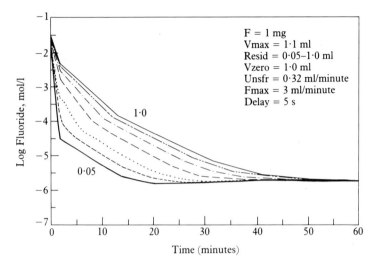

Fig. 3 Effect of the residual volume after swallowing on the clearance process in a computer simulation. Only the residual volume after swallowing is varied, all others factors are kept constant.

the lowest residual volume and the highest volume tested was more than 100-fold after only a few minutes.

The clearance curves show that fluoride concentration declines rapidly during the first minutes. The curve then smoothly adapts to the basal level of the salivary fluoride concentration. This smooth adaptation is caused by the redistribution of fluoride between the plaque (or teeth) and the saliva.

But how does the computer model compare to real life? Figure 4 shows a very similar curve from a study in human subjects after chewing a fluoride-containing chewing gum. The resemblance to the computer-generated curve is remarkable.

Volume of saliva in the mouth just prior to swallowing (maximum volume)

Another important physiological variable affecting salivary clearance is the maximum volume of saliva. The mean volume is 1·1 ml, but like residual volume, a wide range of variation is found in normal individuals.

The effect of this variable on salivary fluoride clearance in the computer model is shown in Figure 5. Again, a large effect on

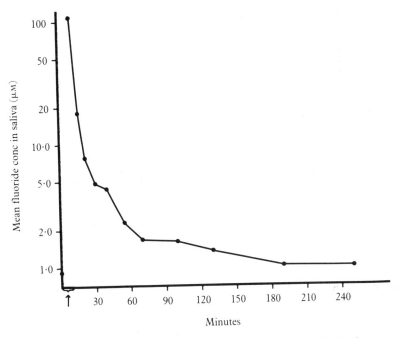

Fig. 4 Salivary clearance of fluoride after intake of 0·25 mg fluoride in a chewing gum.

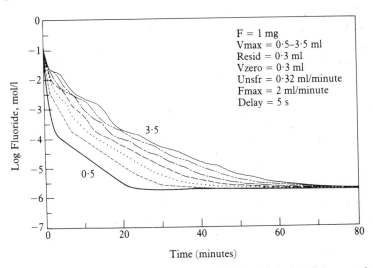

Fig. 5 Effect of the maximum volume before swallowing on the clearance process in a computer simulation.

clearance is seen, and it seems likely, even without clinical evidence, that a variable with such great effects on salivary clearance must be important to oral health.

Unstimulated salivary flow rate

Since the clearance rate is dependent on the entry into the mouth of saliva, it is obvious that the salivary flow rate is an important variable. The unstimulated salivary flow rate is normally about 0·3 ml/minute but may vary a great deal between individuals.

As might be expected, according to our model, varying the unstimulated salivary flow rate has a great effect on fluoride clearance (fig. 6).

The current view of fluoride's role in demineralisation and remineralisation stresses the importance of raising the fluoride levels in the liquid surrounding the enamel crystals for prolonged periods of time. Only a small increase in fluoride (say, from 0·02 to 0·05 or 0·1 ppm) is needed to have a dramatic change in remineralisation provided it can be maintained continually. Factors influencing salivary clearance have an important role in the cariostatic effect of fluoride.

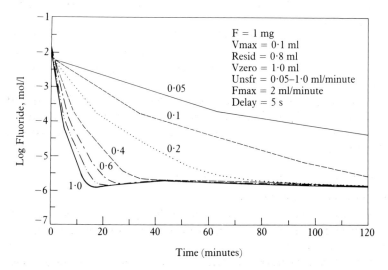

Fig. 6 Effect of the unstimulated salivary flow rate on the clearance process in a computer simulation.

Stimulated salivary flow rate

After a sucrose mouthrinse, this is of little importance in oral clearance, since the stimulus to salivation from rinsing is small and persists only for a very short period of time. With more normal stimuli such as food or chewing gum, however, it can vary a great deal according to the type of stimulus. It also can have a great effect on the clearance pattern of fluoride on the computer model. In the first part of the clearance curve the effect is very large, even within fairly small levels of stimulation. The faster clearance rate caused by a stimulation of salivary flow reduces the diffusion of fluoride into the dental plaque.

There are no *in vivo* data on this effect yet, but these results suggest that the stimulated flow rate may have great effects on the availability of fluoride to the tooth mineral. In formulating cariostatic topical fluoride products, it thus seems advisable to aim for an agent which does not stimulate salivation, in other words is tasteless. However, stimulation of saliva may be of benefit in distributing fluoride (at low concentrations) around the mouth.

Clearance of substances from local sites

Saliva covers the oral surfaces in a thin film approximately 0·1 mm thick. The rate of flow in different areas affects salivary clearance from different regions of the mouth.

A study compared sucrose clearance after a sucrose mouth-rinse at four sites with that of the bulk saliva (fig. 7). A much slower clearance was found from between the upper centrals compared to between the lower centrals.

When the clearance of sugar from the lower incisor site is measured in different individuals against the measured salivary flow rate, a correlation is seen between the salivary flow rate and individual clearance patterns.

Clearance of substances important to oral health

Clearance of carbohydrates

Dental caries is caused by the demineralising effects of organic acids produced in the plaque by micro-organisms that ferment carbohydrates, most notably sucrose.

Several investigators have tried to establish a correlation between sugar clearance and dental caries, but only a very few of these studies have found a significant correlation. This might be expected, since

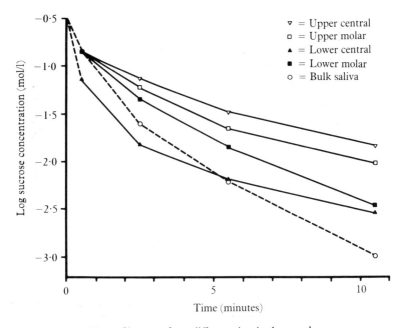

Fig. 7 Clearance from different sites in the mouth.

dental caries is a multifactorial disease, and it is unlikely that a single factor would be decisive.

However, indirectly, the importance of carbohydrate clearance may be shown by its influence on pH. Figure 8 shows the clearance of sucrose and the subsequent pH changes in dental plaque from two subjects, one with fast clearance of sucrose and the other with slow clearance. We found that at a slower clearance rate pH was depressed to a greater degree than at a faster rate. Sucrose concentrations in the early phase of clearance were also significantly correlated to pH in the latter phase of the Stephan curve. Thus a slower clearance rate not only depresses pH but also retards its recovery to the resting value.

Clearance of chloride

In Sweden, as in many other countries, there has been much discussion about the possible adverse effects of amalgam. It is known that amalgams can corrode in the oral environment, and it has been suggested that this can release mercury and other ions with toxic effects. It is also known that chloride has a corroding effect on metals.

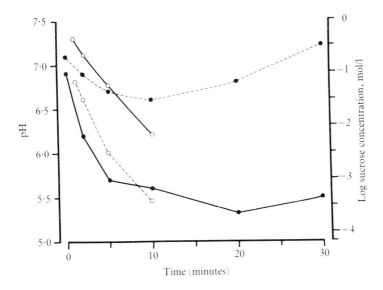

Fig. 8 Effect of sucrose clearance on plaque pH in a subject with fast sucrose clearance (···) and a subject with slow clearance (——).

In an experiment we found that the current density in two half cells containing gold and amalgam showed a correlation with the concentration of sodium chloride in saliva. Normally, the chloride concentration in the salivary secretion is low, approximately 20 mmol/l. However, after ingestion of salty foods, the concentration of chloride can reach very high levels. We therefore decided to test the clearance pattern of chloride.

We found that chloride showed a very similar clearance pattern to that of fluoride, but cleared much more quickly. Individual variation is large, but we do not know yet whether this variation would be significant enough to affect individual corrosion rates of mercury amalgams.

Clearance of chlorhexidine

Chlorhexidine is of course used in dentistry to control infection, especially in the form of rinse solutions or gels for plaque control, to prevent both dental caries and periodontitis.

A feature of chlorhexidine is its adherence to the oral surfaces which gives it a special clearance pattern, and it can remain elevated for many hours.

Conclusion

The clearance pattern of a substance is very important, when trying to estimate the oral bio-availability of a specific substance. There are many factors involved, and clearance patterns for substances like sucrose, fluoride, chloride and chlorhexidine are quite dissimilar. Individual variation in clearance patterns can be both harmful and beneficial. For example, in one study of plaque pH after a bicarbonate rinse, normal subjects showed a rapid rise in pH followed by a rapid fall towards the resting value. In xerostomic patients, however, the pH did not fall back for two hours, presumably causing enhancement of remineralisation during this prolonged time.

Points from the general discussion
The effect of a water mouthrinse on plaque pH

It has often been reported that rinsing the mouth with water after eating or drinking sugary items does not significantly reduce the fall in plaque pH, suggesting perhaps that the role of clearance of sugar (and of plaque acid) by diffusion into a large volume of saliva was overestimated. By contrast, rinsing with a bicarbonate solution was immediately effective in restoring plaque pH, similar to the effect of stimulating saliva. So perhaps the salivary effect was due to the buffering due to bicarbonate in saliva, and not to enhanced clearance.

Mouthrinsing after a sugar challenge does not markedly affect the content of organic acids and of amino acids in plaque, whereas chewing paraffin wax has a dramatic effect. This may reflect not only neutralisation and buffering by bicarbonate, but also the supply of nitrogenous compounds for base production.

The lack of effect of mouthrinsing may be because it is done too late. Two minutes after a sucrose challenge the sugar concentration in saliva is lower than that in plaque, so rinsing would not be expected to accelerate diffusion markedly, unless the sugar clearance is excessively slow as in the case of xerostomic subjects. As far as the removal of acid is concerned, outward diffusion may not adequately explain plaque neutralisation, as protons (H^+ ions) responsible for the low pH are fixed to bacterial proteins and other fixed buffers in plaque. This is why mobile salivary buffers like bicarbonate are so important—they are able to diffuse in, capture the protons from the fixed buffers, and remove them.

Fluoride in saliva

The fluoride level in saliva is seen increasingly as an important measurement to assess the de- and remineralisation potential of the oral cavity. These levels are dominated by exposure to fluoride from dentifrices and other preventive applications. Most studies have failed to demonstrate a relationship between salivary fluoride levels and water fluoride, although some positive results have been observed in British studies.

Summary—Clinical Highlights

- Rapid oral clearance of sucrose and other carbohydrate substrates (and of acid from plaque metabolism) will be of clinical benefit. However, for protective agents like fluoride or chlorhexidine, a slow clearance is preferable. Understanding of the factors determining clearance rate is leading to a more detailed picture of how to maximise benefits—for example, the avoidance of salivary stimulation with fluoride applications.

Further reading

Aasenden R, Brudevold F, Richardson B. Clearance of fluoride from the mouth after topical treatment or the use of a fluoride mouthrinse. *Archs Oral Biol* 1968; **13**: 625–636.

Bibby B G, Mundorff S A, Zero D T, Almekinder K J. Oral food clearance and the pH of plaque and saliva. *J Am Dent Assoc* 1986; **112**: 333–337.

Britse A, Lagerlöf F. The diluting effect of saliva on the sucrose concentration in different parts of the human mouth after a mouthrinse with sucrose. *Archs Oral Biol* 1987; **32**: 755–756.

Dawes C. A mathematical model of salivary clearance of sugar from the oral cavity. *Caries Res* 1983; **17**: 321–334.

Dawes C. Physiological factors affecting salivary flow rate, oral sugar clearance, and the sensation of dry mouth in man. *J Dent Res* 1987; **66**: 648–653.

Ekstrand J, Lagerlöf F, Oliveby A. Some aspects of the kinetics of fluoride in saliva. *In* S A Leach (ed.) *Factors relating to demineralisation and remineralisation of the teeth.* pp 91–98. Oxford: IRL Press, 1986.

Lagerlöf F, Dawes C. The volume of saliva in the mouth before and after swallowing. *J Dent Res* 1984; **63**: 618–621.

Lagerlöf F, Oliveby A, Ekstrand J. Physiological factors influencing salivary clearance of sugar and fluoride. *J Dent Res* 1987; **66:** 430–435.

Lindfors B, Lagerlöf F. Effect of sucrose concentration in saliva after a sucrose rinse on the hydronium ion concentration in dental plaque. *Caries Res* 1988; **22:** 7–10.

Oliveby A, Ekstrand J, Lagerlöf F. Effect of salivary flow rate on salivary fluoride clearance after use of a fluoride containing chewing gum. *Caries Res* 1987; **21:** 393–401.

Swenander-Lanke L. Influences on salivary sugar of certain properties of foodstuffs and individual oral conditions. *Acta Odontol Scand* 1957; **15:** Supplement 23.

Weatherell J A, Strong M, Robinson C, Ralph J P. Fluoride distribution in the mouth after fluoride rinsing. *Caries Res* 1986; **20:** 111–119.

Weatherell J A, Duggal M S, Robinson C, Curzon M E. Site-specific differences in human dental plaque pH after sucrose rinsing. *Arch Oral Biol* 1988; **33:** 871–873.

8

Treatment of Salivary Hypofunctions

Symptoms of dry mouth can be reduced by use of artificial salivas with appropriate lubricant functions. Current work is directed towards increasing the output of any residual gland tissue present.

There are two basic approaches to the treatment of salivary gland hypofunction: intrinsic, exploiting any functional gland present, and extrinsic, involving salivary replacement therapy.

The intrinsic approach

This depends on the presence of functional salivary gland parenchyma, and the ways in which this can be assessed are discussed on pages 92–93.

Once the presence of functioning salivary tissue has been established, there are various strategies open. One of these is to increase dietary bulk and certainly this is an effective tactic in increasing salivation in hypofunctioning rats, although more complete studies have yet to be done in humans.

This discussion will, however, concentrate on the future for genetic regulation of salivary gland function. This involves the use of gene-specific activators, called 'trans-acting factors'. The strategy envisaged would employ trans-acting factors to activate specifically the genes of the residual secretory epithelium of the salivary glands, causing them to proliferate.

In order to be able to appreciate how this might be achieved, it is necessary first to describe the functioning of genes, and their control.

An introduction to molecular genetics

Figure 1 shows a typical gene from a higher organism (eukaryote). It is a stretch of deoxyribonucleic acid (DNA). DNA contains in code form all of the blueprint to make us what we are, the so-called

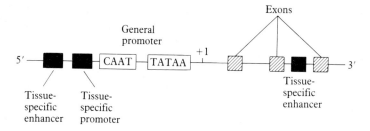

Fig. 1 Diagram of a eukaryotic gene.

genome. Within this stretch of DNA, there are segments called exons, which encode the amino acid sequences for all the protein molecules in the body.

In the lower forms of life, prokaryotes, the coding in DNA is continuous. But in eukaryotes other segments of DNA are found between the exon segments. These intervening segments are called introns. They do not encode information that, as with the exons, is ultimately transcribed by the cell into proteins. This is not to imply, however, that introns are unimportant or redundant.

When a cell manufactures proteins, the DNA in the nucleus is first transcribed, the code is passed on to a molecule of ribonucleic acid RNA. The 5' region is said to be 'upstream', while the 3' region is 'downstream'. When a cell makes a particular protein from this gene, transcription is begun by an enzyme called RNA polymerase which binds to the start site on the gene (part of the intron segment upstream of the gene).

Using the information encoded on the exon segment, the polymerase enzyme transcribes the DNA to form a molecule called messenger RNA. The message delivered by this RNA to the ribosome (the unit of protein synthesis within the cell) is the code for the exact sequence of amino acids required to make up the protein.

Control of gene transcription

Upstream of the start site, there are other specialised regions of DNA called promotor regions. These regions are target sites for regulator proteins, which bind to these regions and speed up the process which transcribes the messenger RNA. Functionally similar to promotors are the enhancers, other segments of the gene which act as target sites and boost the system. Promotors are differentiated from enhancers by their position on the gene—this must always be upstream of the start site. But both promotors and enhancers can speed up transcription of the gene, thereby increasing the amount of messenger RNA and in many instances the final amount of protein produced.

Promotor regions for related genes seem to share common nucleotide sequences. This has been clearly shown for nine different exocrine pancreatic genes. Analysis of their promotor regions showed that there were pancreatic-specific stretches of DNA common to all the genes. If a similar tissue-specific DNA stretch could be identified for the salivary glands, this would enable researchers to develop ways of genetically manipulating the salivary glands—once this salivary gland sequence had been identified, protein analogues could be developed to increase the rate of transcription by areas of these promotor regions. Some of the salivary proteins are uniquely produced in the acinar cells of the submandibular gland, and nowhere else in the body. It may thus be possible to identify and manipulate the genes for these tissue-specific proteins, by regulating their tissue-specific promotors. Thus, one could design a treatment for genetic manipulation.

Other factors which activate genes

Trans-acting factors are proteins which regulate genes. They are thought to work by interlocking with specific stretches of DNA, boosting the transcriptional system so that more protein is made.

Inducible enhancers of transcription include many molecules, such as intracellular messengers, growth factors, and hormones. For example, cyclic AMP (a second messenger in the salivary secretory mechanism, as described on page 101) can also act at a nuclear level to regulate transcription, so too can the intracellular calcium second messenger system. These findings suggest that there is a coupling of gene expression with secretion. This explains why secretory activity increases the rate of synthesis of secretory proteins in salivary acinar cells.

For example, if submandibular gland tissue in one rat is injected with saline, and in another rat, with isoproterenol (a drug which mimicks beta-adrenergic actions including protein secretion), histological examination of the glands shows hyperplasia and hypertrophy (fig. 2) in the rat injected with isoproterenol.

Another experiment with isoproterenol has shown that the drug can induce expression of cystatins, a family of proteins which act as

Control   Isoproterenol

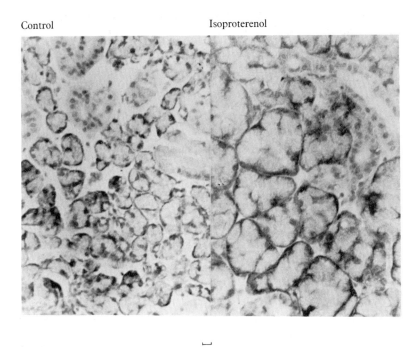

10 μm

Untreated

Fig. 2 Hyperplasia/hypertrophy in rat submandibular salivary glands after injection of
isoproterenol or saline (control).

protease inhibitors. So not only can this secretory drug induce
hyperplasia and hypertrophy of glandular tissue, but it can also turn
on the specific expression of a particular group of proteins.

If we are to be able to manipulate gene expression at the level of
promotors or transactive factors, it will be necessary to deliver them
to the cells. One possible route would be via retrograde perfusion of
the ducts. However, there is a need for much experimental work
before this ideal—of boosting intrinsic tissues by genetically active
drugs—can be achieved.

Extrinsic replacement therapy
It is only in the last few years that enough has been discovered about
normal salivary gland function to begin to define rational approaches
to replacement therapy—the use of 'artificial salivas'.

Two things must be borne in mind. First, that 'saliva is good for you'. So an excellent place to start, if we are to formulate an artificial saliva, is to investigate thoroughly important functions of the fluid.

- *Stimulated saliva acts mainly to flush out the oral environment* by its continued posterior movement towards the back of the mouth where it is finally swallowed.
- *Saliva has a tissue-coating function*, but it is difficult to define what exactly 'lubrication' means.
- *Saliva is important at the interface between the soft tissues and prostheses.* A typical patient complaining of dry mouth often has several sets of dentures that don't fit.
- *Saliva modulates the oral flora* by promoting the selective adhesion and proliferation of micro-organisms. It also has antimicrobial properties against some bacteria, while being used as a metabolic substrate by others.
- *Salivary secretions also have buffering capacity* or are involved in base formation.
- *Saliva may also neutralise potentially deleterious compounds.* There is evidence to show that proline-rich proteins complex tannins, found in many foods, such as celery.
- *Saliva helps stabilise the calcium phosphate equilibrium* involved in the demineralisation and remineralisation of teeth.
- *Saliva dissolves tastants* and transports them to the tastebuds.
- *Saliva aids digestion* by neutralising oesophageal contents and diluting gastric chyme. Salivary amylase helps digestion of large starchy meals.

Secondly, that 'a little goes a long way'. Some people, when speaking about replacement therapy, envisage having to make gallons of artificial saliva, which would be too expensive to be feasible. Yet it is likely that just like the natural substance, very little will suffice.

There is a wide range of salivary output compatible with oral comfort. This includes those with a diminished salivary flow but whose oral mucosal integrity is relatively well maintained.

Role of minor mucous glands

The term 'minor' is a misnomer. It refers only to anatomical size, but they are arguably the most important salivary glands. They are responsible for enveloping all the hard and soft tissues with a thin coat of saliva. These glands supply many important substances to whole saliva, such as most of the blood-group substances (high molecular-weight mucin glycoproteins), immunoglobulins, and other defence proteins.

The characteristic properties of mucin

Mucins are high molecular weight glycoproteins with some unique physicochemical properties. Due to their high content of carbohydrate (70–80%) and complex formation between different polypeptide chains, mucin subunits can stick together. If there is enough mucin, a gelatinous matrix forms which is important in protecting the mouth.

The peculiar physicochemical properties of mucins in saliva are referred to as rheological properties. They include low solubility, high viscosity, high elasticity, and strong adhesiveness. Research has now begun into the correlation between these rheological properties and what makes the mouth 'feel good'.

Viscosity

Research has shown that viscosity differs between unstimulated and stimulated parotid saliva. But more interestingly, if parotid saliva, either unstimulated or stimulated, is freeze-dried and then reconstituted to its original protein weight:volume ratio, this will greatly lower its viscosity. This suggests that somehow a macromolecular complex important to viscosity has been destroyed. A similar result is found with submandibular saliva.

However, replacement therapy using a saliva substance of high viscosity is not sufficient to relieve salivary hypofunction. All the commercially available salivary substitutes tested have been found to have higher viscosities than saliva, but their efficacy is rather limited, and many patients do not like them.

Lubrication

Some years ago researchers devised a friction-testing device to test the abilities of different solutions to reduce frictional drag. In the same way as a needle plays on the surface of a record, so the facial surface of a canine tooth plays on a metal platter. The substance to be tested is interposed between the tooth surface and the platter.

A series of measurements were made of saliva and its components.

Whole submandibular saliva reduced frictional drag well, but mucins had the best lubricating ability. Other salivary glycoproteins were tested, such as the proline-rich proteins, and these also had some lubricating ability.

However this friction-testing device is testing hard surface-to-hard surface contact. This is a good way of studying the lubrication between the teeth in mastication, but the most important lubricatory effects arise from soft tissue-to-soft tissue contacts, or from tooth-to-soft tissue contacts.

So researchers designed another device to study this type of contact. It consists of a turntable, which is mounted and can be positioned in three dimensions using laser beams, with a hard surface made of marble, and a soft surface made of Agarose gel.

Using this model, the frictional coefficients of different oils, distilled water, and different salivary secretions were measured. It was found that water and saliva had similar frictional coefficients, indicating it would seem that saliva is a poor lubricant.

This result could mean two things. The first is that the assay is unsuitable, (and this is under investigation), or second that lubrication in an engineering sense is not the quality we should be trying to study in an artificial saliva. This latter option is favoured, and it is believed that tissue-coating function would be a better description and more useful in formulating a picture of how saliva works in facilitating soft tissue movement.

This property is related to the special rheological characteristics of mucins—their ability to form a gel, their elasticity and adhesiveness. Water-retention by mucosal surfaces is very important and is favoured by mucins, (especially by one type called MG1).

Conclusion

Most of the saliva substitutes currently available are unsuccessful (one available substitute contains sucrose!). The most successful so far is based on mucin, but even so its acceptability is limited. For the future, very basic studies are still needed on the relationship between the structure of saliva and its functions. Once these are more clearly defined, it should be possible to take advantage of biotechnology to prepare sufficient quantities of suitable substances for use in saliva substitutes.

Summary—Clinical Highlights

- Research in molecular biology is poised to discover the mechanisms controlling salivary acinar cell proliferation and gene expression. There is a real possibility that methods will be available to increase specifically the number and activity of gland cells.

- Meanwhile, artificial saliva substitutes have not been successful because the properties which patients need have not been adequately defined or studied.

Further reading

Edgerton M, Tabak L A, Levine M J. Saliva: a significant factor in removable prosthodontic treatment. *J Prosth Dent* 1987; **57:** 57–66.

Levine M J, Aguirre A, Hatton M N, Tabak L A. Artificial salivas: present and future. *J Dent Res* 1987; **66:** 693–698

Mandel I D. The functions of saliva. *J Dent Res* 1987; **66:** 623–627.

Tabak L A, Bowen W H. Roles of saliva (pellicle), diet, and nutrition on plaque formation. *J Dent Res* 1989; 68: 1560–1566.

Tabak L A, Levine M J, Mandel I D, Ellison J A. Role of salivary mucins in the protection of the oral cavity. *J Oral Pathol* 1982; **11:** 1–17.

9

Xerostomia

Xerostomia is an increasingly common clinical condition with a variety of causes; major ones being medication (especially antidepressants), head and neck irradiation, and auto-immune disease, for example Sjögren's syndrome. Drugs stimulating gland function, for example pilocarpine, may have a role in treatment of xerostomia and its sequelae. Xerostomia is the subjective complaint of oral dryness, which may or may not be related to salivary gland dysfunction.

Epidemiology

There are very few epidemiological data on xerostomia. A recent study of the general adult population in Rochester, New York, found a low prevalence, about 2%, in normal healthy individuals. This figure increased to 20%, however, in individuals on medication.

Xerostomia is likely to become even more common as the population in the developed world shifts towards older people. The elderly experience more frequently the iatrogenic and systemic causes associated with xerostomia.

Aetiology

Although a complaint of xerostomia most frequently means that the salivary glands are not working properly this is not always so. The perception of oral dryness can also be the result of a sensory or cognitive disorder. Objective measurements may show that a patient has normal salivary flow but his mouth still 'feels dry'. In addition, changes in salivary composition separate from flow rate may result in complaints of dryness.

Sequelae (Table 1)

Individuals with true salivary gland hypofunction will have considerable discomfort, inconvenience and a diminished quality of life. They are more susceptible to caries and mucosal changes (for example ulceration and candida infection). Patients who have some

Table 1 Local and systemic conditions associated with a dry mouth

Oral	Systemic
Caries	Associated with a number of fatal or
Mucosal ulceration	morbid disorders (for example malig-
Infections (for example candida)	nant lymphoma, polyglandular failure
Difficulty with mastication,	syndrome, primary biliary cirrhosis,
swallowing and taste	polymyositis)

gland function remaining often add to their problems by sucking sweets, especially fruit-flavoured boiled sweets which are themselves acidic, in order to stimulate salivary flow. Conversely, stimulation of saliva by chewing a sugar-free gum or candy could be of benefit by increasing salivary flow and the potential for remineralisation of early lesions. Problems of caries can be treated at home by the use of fluoride—for example, a 1% gel or 0·05% sodium fluoride rinse twice daily.

Taste may also be affected. Saliva does not seem to play a direct role in maintaining the function of the taste-buds, but it is necessary to dissolve and transport taste substances to the taste-buds. The mastication and swallowing of food is also impaired.

Systemically, inadequate saliva is also a sign associated with several morbid or fatal disorders, mostly auto-immune. For example, the incidence of malignant lymphoma in patients with Sjögren's syndrome, an auto-immune exocrinopathy and the single most common systemic cause of reduced salivary gland function, is 40–60 times that of age- and sex-matched controls. So the complaint of oral dryness is not a trivial one and deserves proper evaluation.

Age and salivary function

Salivary gland hypofunction is not a normal part of growing old. However, it is associated with situations that are commoner in middle age and older individuals. A study done several years ago (Table 2) found age made no statistically significant difference to an individual's ability to make parotid saliva, either stimulated or unstimulated. These findings are supported by a more recent study, which found no significant change in the output of stimulated or unstimulated submandibular saliva in healthy individuals across the lifespan. Patients' sensitivity to taste, smell, heat, texture, and viscosity appear

Table 2 Ageing and parotid salivary function in males[a]

	Young (<39 years)	Middle-aged (40–59 years)	Old (>60 years)
Unstimulated (ml/minute)	0·056	0·047	0·044
Stimulated (ml/minute)	0·800	0·619	0·843

[a] Data modified from Heft and Baum, *J Dent Res* 1984; **63**: 1182.

not to be reduced with increasing age (although tactile pressure sensitivity is). So the major components of the input for the gustatory reflex remain active in healthy older people.

Evaluation of 'dry mouth'

Patients presenting with a complaint of xerostomia require a careful evaluation. A detailed history of symptoms and a physical evaluation, including oral, general and serological assessments should be obtained. Gland function should be assessed as well as related functions, such as swallowing. It has been found that subjective responses by patients to four questions can greatly aid diagnosis (Table 3). Patients who respond positively are very likely to have salivary gland hypofunction.

Detection of Sjögren's syndrome

When Sjögren's syndrome is suspected a labial biopsy should be performed. This involves clamping the lower lip making a small incision, and excising minor mucous salivary glands. They are then examined histologically by a pathologist for periductular lymphocytic focal infiltration (fig. 1)—evidence of Sjögren's syndrome. Nine times as many women, mostly postmenopausal, have Sjögren's syndrome as men. In primary Sjögren's, there is no associated connective tissue disorder.

Table 3 Questionnaire to identify dry mouth

Do you sip liquids to aid swallowing dry food?
Does your mouth feel dry when you eat a meal?
Do you have difficulty in swallowing any foods?
Does the amount of saliva in your mouth seem too little rather than too much?

Modified from Fox *et al.*, *J Amer Dent Ass* 1987; **115**: 381.

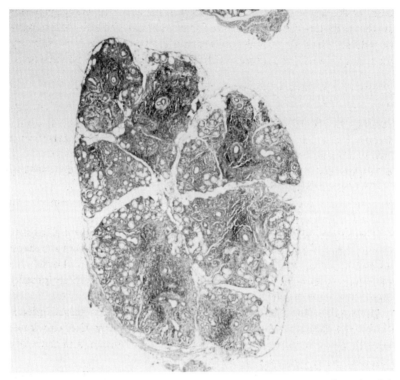

Fig. 1 Minor labial gland biopsy from Sjögren's syndrome (Haematoxylin and eosin). showing multiple foci of lymphocytic infiltration.

Assessing the presence of functioning glandular epithelium

Technetium pertechnate uptake

A useful tool to assess gland function is salivary scintigraphic scanning. The radioisotope used is technetium pertechnate (^{99m}Tc), a gamma emitter with a short half-life of 6 hours. It is taken up by acinar cells in the salivary glands, as well as by cells in the thyroid and gastrointestinal tract.

Technetium pertechnate enters the salivary gland acinar cells via the $Na^+/K^+/Cl^-$ co-transporter mechanism which is the main way chloride ions enter the acinar cells against a steep electrochemical gradient (see p. 103). The movement of chloride ions across acinar cells is the key event in saliva production, and this co-transporter system provides the driving force for secretion of the fluid component of saliva. Thus the uptake of technetium pertechnate by salivary glands indicates the presence of functional glandular epithelial cells.

Responders or non-responders

A quick and convenient screening test, suitable for use in a clinical setting has been developed by workers in the Dental School at Stony Brook, USA. Patients complaining of dry mouth are categorised into two groups according to their ability to secrete whole saliva:

- responders—patients in whom it is possible to stimulate salivary flow by swabbing the tongue with 2% citric acid
- non-responders—patients who don't secrete saliva in response to the stimulus.

This simple test can avoid the initial need for salivary scintigraphy. General practitioners can carry it out in the surgery with a swab soaked in 2% citric acid, and a graduated tube to measure the volume of saliva spat out. However, to determine therapy, scintigraphy should be carried out.

Responders by definition have functional salivary gland epithelium, with a functioning $Na^+/K^+/Cl^-$ co-transporter that can move choride or technetium across the acinar cell membrane, and therefore can also move water across the acinar cell.

Non-responders probably have no functional epithelium, and thus cannot handle technetium pertechnate correctly. They have defective or absent acinar cells, and therefore cannot move fluid, and so will not respond to drug treatment to stimulate salivary secretions. These patients will need salivary subsitutes, which unfortunately at present are not wholly satisfactory.

Medical management of xerostomia

'Responders', as defined above, may be good candidates for treatment with a sialogogue. The use of low doses of orally administered pilocarpine (a parasympathomimetic drug) has been particularly successful in this regard.

Candidate patients require extensive testing of salivary function. They must be in good general health, for although pilocarpine is a drug that stimulates salivary flow it may also have systemic effects. With careful evaluation, patients can be selected with enough functional acinar epithelial cells to warrant pilocarpine treatment.

Clinical studies of the use of pilocarpine

A study published in 1986 by researchers at NIDR investigated the use of pilocarpine in six patients with Sjögren's syndrome or chronic non-specific sialadenitis. They were all female, aged between 62–76 years, and had complained of oral dryness for varying periods up to 10 years at the most. They all had no, or little, unstimulated secretion, but had the ability to respond to a citric acid stimulus, that is they were 'responders', and their Technetium pertechnate scans showed some uptake although little or no basal release.

These patients were given pilocarpine or placebo in a double-blind crossover study. Pilocarpine was chosen because it is a well-characterised drug, and it has been known for many years that it stimulates salivary flow by binding to muscarinic receptors on acinar cell surfaces. Each patient took placebo for 2 days followed by pilocarpine, 5 mg by mouth for 2 days (or vice versa). The results showed a good secretory response similar to that with 2% citric acid on the days that pilocarpine had been taken (fig. 2). A second study was carried out to evaluate a slow release tablet, also 5 mg, held in the mouth. However this method of delivery seemed no more efficacious than ingesting a single oral dose of pilocarpine.

A recent study of the therapeutic use of pilocarpine, just completed, has investigated the effect of giving 5 mg of pilocarpine by mouth 3 times daily. In a 6-month double-blind trial, patients were given 5 mg of pilocarpine at 8 am, 1 pm, and 6 pm each day for 5 months. They were given placebo for one randomised month of the trial period (not the first month).

The patients were seen monthly during treatment. At each visit, unstimulated parotid and submandibular saliva was collected, and their heart rate, blood pressure and ECG were measured. Patients also kept daily diaries of their subjective impressions.

In terms of subjective results, 27 out of the 31 patients who completed the study (87%) noted an improvement varying from pronounced (6 patients) to moderate (14 patients) or minimal (7 patients). The most common comments were decreased oral dryness and improved chewing and swallowing. Side-effects (for example sweating, lacrimation and the urge to urinate) were mild and easily tolerated. There were no significant changes in heart rate, blood pressure, or ECG.

Despite the side-effects experienced, all 31 individuals wished to continue with pilocarpine therapy. Objective measurements of saliv-

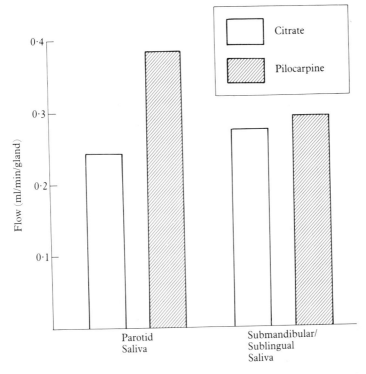

Fig. 2 Saliva response to pilocarpine.

ary output found an increase in unstimulated flow (that is without citric acid) in 75% of the patients.

To summarise, experience shows that it is possible to manipulate hypofunctioning salivary gland cells so that they secrete at reasonable levels; reasonable is defined subjectively by the individual patient.

However, it is important to remember that this drug therapy (pilocarpine) is only one possible treatment, other regimes may be more appropriate for other types of dysfunction, and new possibilities require development and testing. Patients with xerostomia, due to the side-effects of medication, are unlikely to be helped by pilocarpine, and should not be adding another to their list of drugs. It would be more appropriate for their drug to be substituted with one without the side-effect of dry mouth. Drug companies have an interest in developing new or modified drugs without the side-effect of xerostomia.

10

Secretory Mechanisms of Saliva and their Manipulation

The activation of molecular mechanisms signalling intracellular secretory events should be the target for new drugs to compensate for xerostomia.

Salivary gland structure

Figure 1 shows a diagrammatic cross section of a salivary gland. The secretory part of the gland is the acinus (figs 2 and 3). It produces both the protein components of saliva, for example amylase or mucin, as well as the fluid and electrolyte components of saliva. Secretion of protein and of fluids are activated by separate mechanisms.

The glands are innervated by both parasympathetic and sympathetic nerve fibres. Different stimuli produce different ratios of parasympathetic to sympathetic activation (Table 1). If sympathetic stimulation predominates, the secretion will contain a greater amount of protein, while a predominantly parasympathetic secretion will be more copious and watery. However, there is considerable interaction between the pathways, both at the nerve endings and later in the mechanisms of secretion.

The salivary fluid secreted by the acini is isotonic. As it passes down the salivary ducts, it becomes more dilute, and eventually reaches the oral cavity as a hypotonic fluid.

Macromolecular secretion

The macromolecular (protein) components of saliva are secreted by a complex process known as stimulus-secretion coupling (fig. 4). This process is triggered by the attachment of a neuro-transmitter to a receptor on the acinar cell membrane. The neuro-transmitters involved in protein secretion are mainly β-adrenergic.

This generates a second messenger, cyclic AMP, which in turn initiates a variety of physiological changes. These are mediated by kinase enzymes, leading to protein phosphorylation, secretory gra-

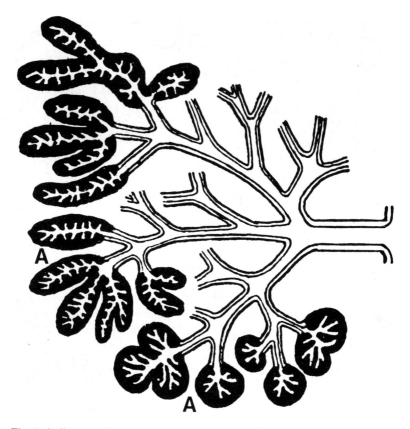

Fig. 1 A diagrammatic section of a salivary gland. This is a typical tubulo-acinar gland. The secretory endpieces (A) release both the macromolecular and fluid components of saliva which are conveyed to the mouth via the branching duct system.

nule movement, and finally exocytosis. These later phenomena are complex, and as this chapter is primarily concerned with manipulating salivary secretion, further discussion will concentrate on the first stage of secretion, since at present this is the only stage which can be manipulated *in vivo*.

The process by which the activation of the receptor by the neurotransmitter leads to activation across the cell membrane of the enzyme which generates the second messenger is called signal transduction.

The key factors in the cyclic AMP signal transduction process are

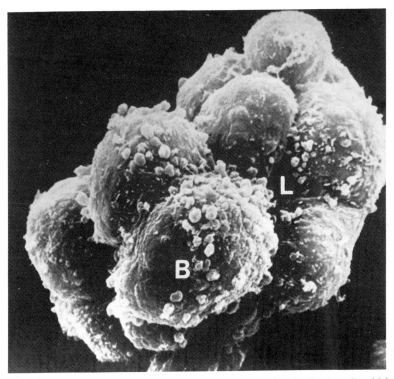

Fig. 2 A scanning electron micrograph of a submandibular gland acinus in which secretory cells are grouped like a bunch of grapes around a central lumen (L) into which the secretory products are released. The surface blebs (B) are preparation artefacts.

Table 1 Control of salivary secretion

Component	Content	Stimulus	Signal transduction
Macromolecular	Mucin Amylase	β-Adrenergic	Adenylate cyclase (cAMP)
Fluid	H_2O electrolytes Na^+, Cl^- and so on	Muscarinic Alpha -ad. Peptidergic	Phosphoinositide effect (IP_3, DG, Ca^{2+})

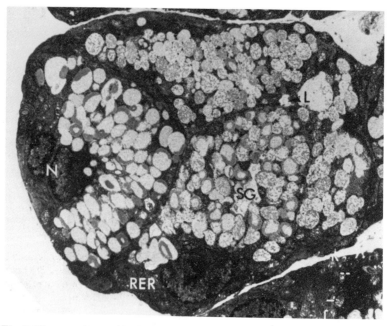

Fig. 3 Electron micrograph of a section of a submandibular gland acinus. The basal area of the cells is occupied by the nucleus (N) and extensive rough endoplasmic reticulum (RER) where the macromolecular secretory product is synthesised. The apical portion of the cells is packed with mucin-containing secretory granules (SG). In the resting state the lumen (L) is narrow.

shown (fig. 5). They include the receptor molecules on the outer face of the cell membrane, regulatory proteins (known as G-proteins) which can be either inhibitory or excitatory, and an effector enzyme adenylate cyclase, which is responsible for converting intracellular ATP to cyclic AMP (the second messenger).

The excitatory neurotransmitters are adrenaline and noradrenaline, while the inhibitory receptors respond to acetylcholine or substance P.

The overall activity of adenylate cyclase probably reflects the balance between stimulatory and inhibitory effects.

Fluid and electrolyte secretion

Again the signal transduction system comprises a receptor, regulatory G-protein, effector enzyme, substrate, and second messenger (fig. 6). In this case, the key molecule is a membrane phospholipid called phosphatidylinositol (4,5)-bisphosphate (PIP_2).

Stimulus-secretion coupling

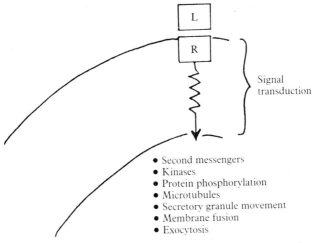

Fig. 4 Stimulus-secretion coupling in salivary gland cells is a complex process requiring many stages to link receptor activation to the exocytotic response. The initial phase of this process is the generation of a second messenger via a series of receptor-coupled reactions in the membrane-signal transduction.

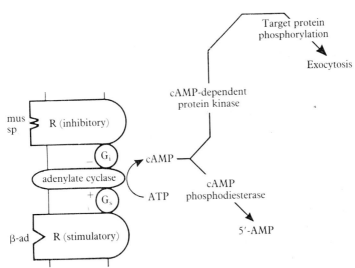

Fig. 5 The major features of the cyclic AMP (cAMP) generating signal transduction system. The enzyme adenylate cyclase is activated via a GS regulatory protein by β-adrenergic stimulation when a suitable neurotransmitter substance (noradrenaline) is released and binds to the receptor. Stimulation of other receptors (for example muscarinic and substance P receptors) cause the coupling of an inhibitory protein (Gi protein) to adenylate cyclase, thus reducing cAMP synthesis.

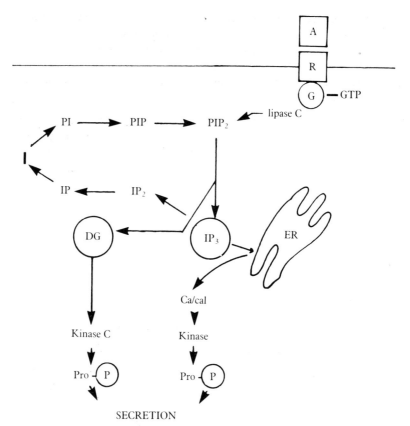

SECRETION

Fig. 6 A simplified outline of the phosphoinositide signal transduction pathway. Stimulation of a receptor (R) by an agonist (A) (for example muscarine, causes activation of the enzyme phospholipase C via a GTP-binding regulatory protein (G). Lipase C cleaves phosphatidylinositol-(4,5) bisphosphate (PIP_2) into two second messengers IP_3 and DG (see text for abbreviations). IP_3 causes the mobilisation of calcium from endoplasmic reticulum stores, which activates kinase enzymes to cause protein phosphorylation and exocytosis. DG may also stimulate secretion by a separate route. The inositol in IP_3 is recycled into PIP_2 in the phosphoinositide cycle.

Binding of neurotransmitter to the receptor and coupling of the G-protein activates an enzyme, phospholipase C. This enzyme hydrolyses PIP_2 to produce two independent second messengers:

● inositol (1,4,5)-trisphosphate (IP_3). IP_3 releases calcium ions from intracellular stores. The elevated calcium ion levels have a variety of intracellular effects, especially triggering a change in membrane permeability to potassium ions thus stimulating their efflux from the cell which is the major process in fluid secretion.

- diacylglycerol (DG) stimulates protein kinase C, which is believed to regulate a Na^+/H^+ exchange mechanism also required for fluid secretion.

As potassium ions leave the cell, the extracellular concentration of potassium ions will increase. This activates a carrier protein ('cotransporter') in the membrane which permits the potassium to re-enter the cell accompanied by Na^+ and Cl^- (fig. 7). This results in an

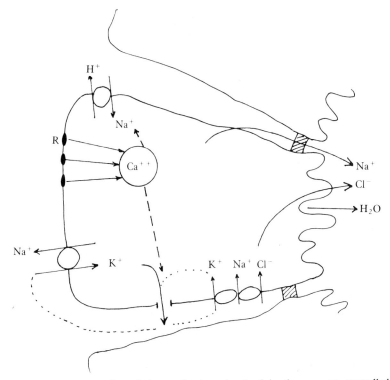

Fig. 7 Simplified outline of the mechanisms involved in the receptor-controlled release of water and electrolytes in salivary gland acinar cells. The initial efflux of K^+ from the cells permits the entry of Na^+ and Cl^- which move through the apical membrane into the lumen and establish an electro-osmotic gradient to stimulate the movement of fluid out of the cells.

increase in intracellular Cl^- ions, which then pass through the apical plasma membrane into the lumen of the acinus. An electro-ionic gradient is set up which draws sodium into the lumen. This means that the sodium chloride concentration becomes higher inside the lumen than outside it, and water flows into the lumen to redress the osmotic imbalance.

Usually, at the same time as water flows into the lumen, secretory granules are discharging their contents, so that the resultant fluid is a complex mixture of water, electrolytes, and macromolecular secretions.

Manipulation of salivary mechanisms in the clinical situation

Knowledge of the mechanisms of salivary secretion can help in the management of abnormal salivary function. Abnormal secretion broadly divides into:

- hypersalivation (sialorrhoea)
- hyposalivation (xerostomia).

Hypersalivation is rare. Occasionally it is reported to occur in conditions when the oesophagus is irritated, such as carcinoma. It may also occur in pregnancy. Drugs to 'dry up' excessive salivation (for example scopolamine) can lead to drowsiness or imbalance, side-effects which are worse problems than the hypersalivation for which they are prescribed. Hyposalivation is the greater problem, and has several causes (see pages 3 and 16).

Knowledge of the stimulus-secretion coupling system should potentially allow intervention to stimulate secretion (fig. 8). Experiments are already being done in isolated salivary gland cells in the laboratory. These mostly involve cells made more permeable to stimulatory agents. This is not feasible in a patient. At present, clinical intervention is only possible at the beginning of the process (that is at the level of the receptor). An example of this is the use of pilocarpine (a muscarinic agonist) for the treatment of xerostomia, as described above (see pages 94–95).

Most of the components involved in stimulus-secretion coupling, or chemicals which may modify their effects, do not readily get inside the cell. Moreover, a chemical agent must be targeted to the salivary acinar cells and not to other cells. In the future, it may be possible to make synthetic drugs which will be site-directed (for example, by

Possible loci of intervention to regulate secretion

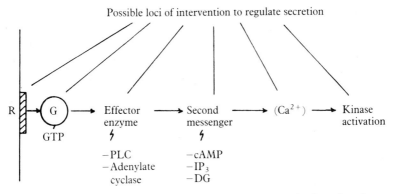

R   G ⟶ Effector ⟶ Second ⟶ (Ca^{2+}) ⟶ Kinase
             enzyme   messenger   activation
   GTP   ⚡   ⚡
           −PLC   −cAMP
           −Adenylate   −IP$_3$
           cyclase   −DG

Fig. 8 Possible loci for intervention to regulate secretory mechanisms in salivary exocrine cells.

being encapsulated in lipid membranes, carried by monoclonal antibodies to attach them to specific cells). A commercial derivative of IP 3 is now available which can cross the cell membrane and (once inside the cell) release IP 3 in its normal active form. This opens up the possibility of using our knowledge of acinar cell physiology to manufacture 'designer drugs' for the benefit of the increasing numbers of patients suffering the discomfort and disease associated with xerostomia.

Points from the general discussion
Salivary function tests in general practice

Experience in the USA has shown that most patients attending dental hospital clinics for dry mouth are referred by physicians (often rheumatologists) for diagnosis of Sjögrens syndrome, and general dental practitioners have little awareness of xerostomia as a clinical problem. This situation is beginning to change, however, and dental schools are teaching the use of salivary function tests.

The main value of these tests is in following change in salivary function, as a careful history and clinical examination can be more useful in diagnosis of xerostomia. However, such tests are relatively rapid and simple, equivalent to taking routine blood pressure measurements, and could be done by a dental auxiliary.

Flow rates are easily measured by asking the patient to spit into a tube over a period of 5 minutes. The volume of saliva can be measured by using a graduated tube, or weighing the tube before and after collection (the density of saliva is very close to 1·0). Collection of the stimulated saliva may present problems because of the small volume, those with dry mouth may not have an unstimulated flow. Stimulated saliva can be elicited by swabbing the tongue with a throat swab moistened with 5% citric acid solution (pure lemon juice may be an acceptable and easily obtained alternative).

Unstimulated flow rates below 0·1 ml/minute, and stimulated flow rates below 0·2 ml/minute, would be regarded as abnormal.

Of the two, measurement of stimulated flow is easier to perform and is advantageous because it will reveal those patients who cannot be helped to increase their salivation (for example by pilocarpine) and who will therefore need to use an artificial saliva.

Patients with low flow rates may not complain of dry mouth symptoms, but their salivary hypofunction may be a cause of poor denture retention or high caries rates. Their salivary function should be monitored in case their glands are subject to progressive pathological change. Those with dry mouth symptoms associated with a normal flow rate do not require treatment of a salivary problem, but their complaint should be further investigated in case it is obscuring a different clinical problem.

The practicality of carrying out salivary function tests will vary from country to country, and between practices. In some circumstances, they will be justified while in others economic considerations will not justify the use of a dentist's time (or that of his assistant). It is important that they do not result in the accumulation of information which is not used; this suggests that practitioners should restrict their use to patients complaining of dry mouth. As far as the NHS in Britain is concerned, it is clear that a detailed cost/benefit analysis would be needed before such tests could be incorporated into routine patient care. However, a plea can be made that general practitioners should be more aware of the prevalence of salivary hypofunction. If 30% of the general adult population have some symptoms associated with dry mouth, tests of salivary function are increasingly likely to feature among the diagnostic procedures available to the dentist.

Summary—Clinical Highlights

- Increased knowledge of the intracellular signalling mechanisms of salivary acinar cells present potential opportunities for manipulating salivary secretion, both of macromolecules and of the fluid phase of saliva.
- Current technology will only permit manipulation at the level of the receptor, but it is only a matter of time—before post-receptor modification of the secretory processes will be possible. For example, at present, polarised molecules cannot cross the membrane. If ways can be found to deliver these agents into the cell, then events at the synthetic level could be manipulated, permitting development of new agonists for highly specific tasks.

Further reading

Baum B J. Neurotransmitter control of secretion. *J Dent Res* 1987; **66:** 628–632.

Fleming N, Bilan P T, Sliwinski-Lis E, Carvalho V. Muscarinic, alpha-1 adrenergic and peptide agonists stimulate phosphoinositide hydrolysis and regulate mucin secretion in rat submandibular gland cells. *Pflugers Arch* 1987; **409:** 416–421.

Martinez J R. Ion transport and water movement. *J Dent Res* 1987; **66:** 638–647.

Michell R H, Drummond A H, Downes C P (eds). *Inositol lipids and cell signalling*. London: Academic Press, 1989.

Naccache P H (ed.). *G proteins and calcium signalling*. Boca Raton: CRC Press, 1990.

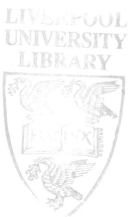